Sophie Fletcher is a clinical hypnotherapist and doula. After gaining a Masters degree in European Culture (specialising in symbolism) from the University of Manchester, she went on to train as a clinical hypnotherapist for pregnancy and birth. Sophie trains midwives in the psychology of birth, is a guest lecturer at Nottingham University School of Midwifery as well as being a fellow of and advisor for the National Council for Hypnotherapy, the leading professional body for hypnotherapy in the UK. Mum of two spirited boys, she divides her time between London and her home in Lincolnshire.

To Jenny, my mother.
Thank you from my heart for being a loving
and compassionate teacher and for your
unending support and advice.

MINDFUL
HYPNO
BIRTHING

Hypnosis and mindfulness techniques
for a calm and confident birth

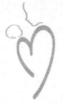

Sophie Fletcher

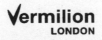
Vermilion
LONDON

9 10 8

Published in 2014 by Vermilion, an imprint of Ebury Publishing
Ebury Publishing is a Random House Group company

Copyright © Sophie Fletcher 2014
Illustrations copyright © Stuart Flockhart 2014

Sophie Fletcher has asserted her right to be identified as the author of this Work
in accordance with the Copyright, Designs and Patents Act 1988

The Random House Group Limited Reg. No. 954009
Addresses for companies within the Random House Group can be found at
www.randomhouse.co.uk

Penguin Random House is committed to a sustainable future for
our business, our readers and our planet. This book is made from
Forest Stewardship Council® certified paper.

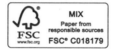

MIX
Paper from
responsible sources
FSC® C018179

Printed and bound in Great Britain by Clays Ltd, St Ives plc

Designed and set by seagulls.net

ISBN 9780091954598

Copies are available at special rates for bulk order. Contact the sales development team
on 02078408487 for more information

To buy books by your favourite authors and register for offers visit
www.randomhouse.co.uk

The information in this book has been compiled by way of general guidance in relation to
the specific subjects addressed, but is not a substitute and not to be relied on for medical,
healthcare, pharmaceutical or other professional advice on specific circumstances and in
specific locations. So far as the author is aware the information given is correct and up to
date as at March 2014. Practice, laws and regulations all change, and the reader should
obtain up to date professional advice on any such issues. The author and publishers
disclaim, as far as the law allows, any liability arising directly or indirectly
from the use, or misuse, of the information contained in this book.

When the ocean surges
Don't let me just hear it.
Let it splash inside my chest!

Rumi

CONTENTS

INTRODUCTION

On Christmas Day in 2003, my first son was born in an operating theatre by Caesarean section. It was my husband and a series of strangers who held him first, while I was dizzy, disorientated and dressed in a hospital gown, unable to walk or hold my baby.

In the following days and weeks, I started suffering from postnatal depression and I found it hard to bond with my son. This was far from the experience of birth and motherhood I had been expecting. Seventeen months later, my second son was born. Even though he was born early, at 32 weeks, I had an undisturbed delivery. I was up straight away, feeling great and able to swing my toddler around. Against the odds, feeding was established early and we left the hospital after just six days. It was liberating, physically and emotionally, and the only difference was the way I had approached the birth.

During my first pregnancy, I didn't really think about the birth. I worked hard in my job until the last minute, felt stressed and worried about all sorts of work-related issues, and had terrible heartburn and intermittent sleep. When I became pregnant with my second son, somehow I knew that this birth would be different. This time I wanted to be in control of what was happening. I did a bit of research and bought myself some hypnosis CDs, which I listened to from early in my pregnancy. I was relaxed, I approached work differently and when my waters broke at 32 weeks I was incredibly calm. Even my husband was surprised at how relaxed his previously highly strung wife was.

I have no doubt that how I approached my birth made a difference to how I birthed. I slept well throughout my pregnancy; I was tuned in to my body; I knew that I could do it, laughing and joking with the midwives instead of worrying about what might go wrong. I'd learned at a deeply subconscious level that by staying calm I was giving my baby the best chance, and the most incredible thing was that it was automatic. I didn't have to 'try' to be calm.

After this birth, my husband, who has a doctorate in bio-chemistry and likes to see evidence, encouraged me to find out more. I trained to be a hypnotherapist, and took courses in several different kinds of hypnosis for birth and the psychology of birth. What I learned was extraordinary: women, like me, were having birth experiences that they described as euphoric, self-affirming and empowering. I wanted other mums-to-be to discover that birth can be different and so much better than they are led to believe.

It's now widely accepted that being relaxed and prepared emotionally can help you have a better birth. Birthing centres everywhere are being redesigned to be more comfortable and homely, and this is a great step forward. However, they don't take account of the unconscious fear that women have about birth, which is a result of dramatic stories and media portrayals of painful, distressing births. Midwives see undisturbed births every day; women do not. We take birth to be what we see on television or what friends and family tell us. Mindful hypnobirthing preparation explores what the unconscious responses around birth can be, how they affect us and what we can do to change our experience to be a better one.

The birthing partner's role is also crucial. My husband was in the dark at my first son's birth, but now the birthing partners I work with – dads, partners, mums, sisters and friends – say how much learning mindful hypnobirthing helped them support the mother during the birth.

There isn't a 'right way' or a 'wrong way' to give birth, but understanding why you choose the birth you do and being mindful of how the birth can affect your baby and your relationship with your baby is extremely important. By trusting your instincts and asking the questions that are important to you, you can take ownership of your birth and feel empowered and confident, whether you are aiming to have a drug-free birth without intervention or a Caesarean.

I want to share with you what I've learned through my study of hypnosis and mindfulness, and my extensive work with women, men and childbirth professionals. Most of all, I want to show you what makes a difference, and how the link between your environment, your body and your baby is crucial. Equipped with the tools and techniques in this book, you'll feel that you are in control and calmly excited about your baby's birth.

HOW TO USE THIS BOOK

Although you can dip in and out of this book, ideally you need to follow it through from the beginning. It's designed to be a practical book, and is packed with tools and techniques that will help you prepare for a mindful hypnobirth, including how to access a set of hypnosis and relaxation tracks to listen to.

You'll find the term 'undisturbed birth' frequently in the book. I use this instead of 'normal birth'. Normal birth can mean something different to every woman, and what is normal for one woman may not be normal for another. Undisturbed birth is allowing birth to take its course without interference.

In the first part of the book, 'Preparation and Pregnancy', I've included information about preparing for a mindful hypnobirth.

In this section are techniques such as visualisation and relaxation, and mindful practices that you will need to get used to before you go into labour.

The second part of the book, 'Birth', takes you through what happens during labour. It will show you how to take what you have learned in your preparation and apply it as your labour progresses.

The third part of the book, 'Welcoming your Baby to the Family', offers practical tips on making those first few days and weeks easier.

Throughout the book you will see this symbol ☺ next to an exercise you can practise. There are tips all the way through from parents who have experienced hypnobirthing. Case studies illustrate some of the important points in the book.

At the very end there is a small selection of birth stories from parents who have used the techniques in this book so you can see how mindful hypnobirthing has made a difference to their births.

You can access three hypnosis tracks at www.mindful-hypnobirthing.co.uk to help you prepare for the birth of your baby. The tracks are to be used alongside the book. The first is a 30 minute deep relaxation track; the second is a series of pregnancy affirmations to help you to adapt to the changes pregnancy brings; and the third is a set of birth affirmations to build your confidence and prepare you for labour. For full details on how and when to listen to them, see page 36.

Have fun exploring. Take what you learn and adapt it as you will, but most of all make it your own.

PART 1
PREPARATION AND PREGNANCY

1

WHAT IS MINDFUL HYPNOBIRTHING?

Childbirth can be made absolutely painless; not only that, it can easily be made pleasurable, ecstatic, under hypnosis.

Osho

Mindful hypnobirthing is a combination of hypnosis and mindfulness techniques. It helps your body respond well during labour by enabling you to create confident, calm and positive thoughts about the birth of your baby. Mums who have used this technique always comment on how they looked forward to the birth of their baby, feeling calmly excited rather than apprehensive or anxious.

Both hypnosis and mindfulness can help you connect with the part of you that is beneath your conscious awareness. This element of mindful hypnobirthing gives you the opportunity to shift your thinking from a state of fear, anxiety or apprehension to calm, confident expectation. Mindful hypnobirthing differs from basic relaxation techniques as it helps change your responses to birth at an unconscious level, which is, ultimately, much more powerful. Using hypnosis to prepare for birth will not only help you during labour and birth but also, potentially, in other areas of your life for many years to come.

HYPNOSIS AND MINDFULNESS

What is Hypnosis?

Hypnosis is a naturally occurring state of mind. We experience it twice a day at least: when we drop off to sleep and when we wake up in the morning. It's that comfortable place when we're not quite awake and not quite asleep, when we are slightly drifting off. Some people say it's a lot like daydreaming. This is also known as an alpha (light hypnosis) or a theta (deep hypnosis) brain state. As a therapy it is remarkable. Sometimes, in as little as one hour, people can move forward into positive states of mind, overcoming phobias, habits and behaviours that may have prevented them from leading a fulfilling life.

My first experience of it came with my second birth. It wasn't until I trained that I saw the extent to which hypnotherapy could help move people into a more positive, happier and life-affirming state of mind quickly and with great effect. I'm the third generation in my family working in a psychological field; my grandfather is a famous forensic psychiatrist and my mother a person-centred counsellor. Hypnotherapy was definitely the trade of choice for me. I found it a very quick and effective therapy for some psychological issues that may have taken longer under the care of a more traditional talking therapist.

When you go into hypnosis you access your unconscious. All the experiences you've had; everything you have been told, seen and heard resides in this area of your mind. In actual fact, our conscious mind can only focus on very small bits of information at any one time. Hypnosis is a goal-driven therapy. When using hypnosis I always ask my clients how they wish to be and we work towards that goal using very specific techniques.

What is Mindfulness?

Mindfulness is different. Rather than focusing on a goal in the future, you are turning your attention to the present. Mindfulness is a way of helping you to relate to your life in awareness, openness and loving kindness. By being mindful of how you experience your life you are able to cultivate a sense of clarity, inner calm and gentle compassion.

Being mindful is about being aware of experience and of being in each moment. It's not as simple as knowing you are eating, washing the dishes or in the shower. Sometimes when we eat, we start thinking about things; we start chatting to our partner or watching television. We know we are eating but our attention is not on the process of eating. If we were to eat mindfully we would be aware of the edge of the knife on the potato as it slices it, the sensation of the potato touching our tongue and of chewing that potato while being aware of the flavour and then swallowing. We may consider where that potato has come from and the many people who have worked to bring that potato to the table. Often our mind wanders when we are doing things that are routine; mindfulness is about bringing your attention to what you are doing. When you are being mindful you are in the present, experiencing being alive and alert to your senses, not dwelling in the past or projecting into the future.

What is the Difference between Mindfulness and Hypnosis?

When you are in mindfulness meditation or using hypnosis you can enter into an alpha or a theta brain state, a naturally occurring altered, yet more focused, state of mind. Whether you are using hypnosis or cultivating mindfulness you are quietening down the chattering part of the mind that sometimes lacks clarity or focus.

Hypnosis is a method of taking us intentionally into a theta brain state, where you can access your unconscious to make changes to a negative or problematic pattern of behaviour by projecting into the future or reframing responses to events in the past. Someone can enter a trance-like, or hypnotic, state by themselves, using breath awareness or self-hypnosis.

The real difference between the two techniques is how we use that state. A mindfulness meditation can turn your attention inwards, bringing yourself into the moment and emptying your mind of thoughts. When experiencing hypnosis you are using that same theta state of mind to focus on a goal, perhaps in the future, or on a previous experience to alter your reaction to that experience. The purpose of hypnosis is to change a negative or obstructive pattern of behaviour, whereas when you are using a mindfulness meditation you are completely in the present, emptying your mind and letting go of thoughts.

Sometimes the outcomes of mindfulness and hypnosis can be very similar. Typically, those using these techniques on a regular basis show reduced anxiety, depression and tension and the ability to manage stress more effectively. Evidence of the benefits of hypnotherapy and mindfulness is now so strong in some fields of medicine that their use is advocated to treat things such as insomnia, irritable bowel syndrome (IBS), anxiety and depression. Both techniques are becoming recognised in mainstream psychological care models for the benefits they bring to our everyday lives.

HYPNOSIS FOR BIRTH

Hypnobirthing: a Modern Invention?

You may be surprised to discover that hypnosis for birth is not a modern invention. In 1858, James Braid – commonly known as the father of hypnotherapy – wrote a paper on inducing a woman early for medical reasons using hypnotherapy. In the 1950s, the Soviet Union gathered the findings of an extensive and successful hypnosis for birth programme, which showed that in 83 per cent of births there was a complete or significant reduction in pain when hypnotherapy was used.

Magonet, a doctor and hypnotherapist in the 1950s, believed that 'the time will come when hypnotherapy in antenatal clinics will be regarded as just as important as carrying out pelvic measurements, blood pressure reading and urine examination'. Although Magonet's vision has not been fulfilled, hypnotherapy has become increasingly recognised in birth preparation. Today, it is more commonly known as hypnobirthing. Over the years, many different methods of hypnosis for birth have evolved, all slightly different in content, delivery, length and design but based on the same philosophy: *If the mother is free of fear and trusts her body to do what it does naturally she can have her best birth possible, sometimes even free of pain.*

Early approaches to hypnosis for birth were about pain management, but now the general philosophy underpinning all these methods is that birth is not something to be feared. Hypnobirthing will build your confidence and help you understand – both consciously and at an instinctive, unconscious, level – that you are able to birth your baby and that you can have a positive experience. This means that when you go into labour, your instinctive responses will be calm excitement and a relaxed body.

Approaches to Hypnosis for Birth

There are two approaches to hypnosis for birth. Whichever approach you decide is for you, you'll find the techniques to support you in this book. The first approach is more traditional, focusing on hypnosis as a pain management tool. Most hypnotherapists will use this approach if they haven't done specific training in the connection between the body and the mind during birth. Many women find these techniques very helpful and they are successful in managing chronic pain. These techniques are also used in what is known as hypno-anaesthesiology, used specifically for operations, minor surgical procedures and dental surgery.

The second approach, and the one more commonly used today for birth, is much more comprehensive and takes on board the wider physiology and psychology around birth. You learn about how thoughts held in your unconscious mind can trigger tension and pain in your body. The focus in this approach is to address the fear you may have of birthing and to allow your body to do what it's designed to do. When this approach works, your body releases its own endorphins, natural painkillers, and you may not have any need for pharmacological pain management techniques.

YOUR CONSCIOUS AND UNCONSCIOUS MIND

Hypnosis and other forms of mind therapies work at a much deeper level than our conscious minds. Your conscious mind is your chattering chimp, the part of your brain that is moving around. It may be thinking of 100 different things in quick succession, but never at one time, and is constantly on the go.

Your unconscious mind is the part of your brain that is processing things out of your immediate awareness. Try this exercise:

As you are reading these words, you are at the same time aware of the colour of the floor, the weight of the book in your hand and any sounds around you. Each time you think of something else you may find that your immediate focus switches to something different. The weight of the book is still there, the sounds are still around you, you just aren't consciously aware of them when you are focused on reading these words.

Your mind is constantly absorbing and filtering messages from the world around you without you even realising. This is called *perception without awareness*. Derren Brown, a well-known hypnotist and illusionist, uses this psychological process to his advantage when he builds up a belief or implants a suggestion into someone's mind before doing a 'mind-reading trick'. We create beliefs, thoughts and feelings based on what we have absorbed throughout our lives, either intentionally or unintentionally.

Imagine that your mind is the British Library; every book that has ever been published is stored in that library under different reference systems. You have a reference system for holidays, for birth, for giving speeches, even for making a cup of tea. It's your own personal user guide for how to operate in the world around you; everything you do checks what is in the reference system to know how to respond. If you were to try and comprehend the magnitude of that library and the information within it at one moment in time, it would be impossible. Your brain can't do it.

Your conscious brain can use the reference systems and retrieve information as and when it needs to, but can only process very small amounts at any one time. This means that many of our responses are automatic and can bypass our conscious thinking brain. Often your body responds without you even having to think about what you are doing. Think about riding a bike, making a cup of tea, brushing your teeth – all these things are automatic learned responses that we don't need to consciously think about when we do them.

Later in the book you will learn why these processes between your brain and your body will have such an impact on how you birth. You'll also learn how to alter and change those reference systems for the better so your automatic physical responses help your labour progress quickly and you stay calm and centred.

What Does Hypnosis Feel like?

You will always be in control when you are in hypnosis. I can't make you cluck like a chicken or eat an onion. Stage hypnosis has done a great disservice to hypnotherapy; it's often a clever manipulation of magic, illusion, psychology and hypnosis, nothing like the hypnotherapy practised by thousands of professional hypnotherapists across the country.

When you are in hypnosis, you will be able to open your eyes at any point you wish. It's an extremely relaxing and comforting form of therapy. When I help with births, I always use a progressive relaxation; this means I guide you into hypnosis by giving you suggestions to relax all the muscles in your body. This is the perfect type of hypnosis to learn for birth – when your muscles are relaxed, calm and working harmoniously, your labour is likely to be much quicker.

Most people are very surprised to feel just how relaxing hypnosis is, and how well their body responds to it. You may feel as if you are aware of everything around you or you may feel as if you have gone to sleep; either is perfect. You may feel heavier and your body sinking down, or you may feel as if you are drifting. Trust that your unconscious will take you into hypnosis in a way that is comfortable and right for you; the more you do it and the more trusting you become of the process, the more deeply relaxed you'll be.

If you feel like it's not working for you, keep going; just allow yourself to let go. Perhaps you need to find somewhere where you feel less self-conscious and more secure. Suddenly it will click and you'll be amazed at just how easy it is to let go and enjoy that deep state of relaxation.

MINDFULNESS FOR BIRTH

Birth can be approached mindfully. It's an opportunity to put aside judgments and expectations and to be aware of the experience of being in the moment with your body and your baby. Jon Kabat-Zinn, an expert in mindfulness and the author of *The Inner Work of Mindful Parenting*, writes: 'Being fully present from one moment to the next during labour requires courage, concentration and the love and support of the people around you.'

Being mindful during your birth is to be connected to the experience and the rhythm of your body in each moment. When you are experiencing the present, you allow yourself to move away from any fears that may rest in the past and back from fears of an imagined future. In the moment, you allow yourself to surrender to the deep trust you have in yourself and your natural abilities to tap into your own inner resources and strength.

Through this awareness of each moment and by being present, we are able to be more in touch with what we need in that moment. Many women who have learned hypnotherapy for birth actually find that staying with their breath and being focused on that breath is all they need. It's this state of mindful awareness that allows you to respond to the needs of your birthing body.

When you stay with your breath, you become focused on your breathing. Try this now:

> Close your eyes and focus on your breathing. Become aware of the coolness of the air as you breathe in, the air expanding your chest. Then be aware of the warmth of the air as you breathe out, your chest falling. Breathing in, coolness, your chest rising; breathing out, warmth, your chest falling. Continue to do this for a few minutes, focusing on the sensations of breathing in and breathing out.

Any sensations you experience during the birth are messages from your body. Turning towards those sensations and embracing them in the moment as something positive – welcoming them, rather than resisting them – will allow your body to let go and open up. This awareness may encourage you to get into different positions or move in a particular way. Being in the moment opens up this connection between your body and your mind and can heighten intuition of how you need to move, rock and sway during labour.

THE PERFECT COMBINATION
FOR A POSITIVE BIRTH

Hypnosis and mindfulness are the perfect combination for a positive birth experience. Your hypnosis preparation will help to process unconscious fears, allowing your body to relax and respond to labour in the way that it is designed to do. Mindfulness will help you be present in each moment during labour. Hypnosis and mindfulness work well in conjunction with other classes you may have attended, such as active birth or pregnancy yoga.

Helping You Stay Centred in your Birthing Zone

Mindful hypnobirthing will teach you how to stay centred in your birthing zone. Your *birthing zone* is a naturally occurring state of mind during birth. If you are free of fear, calmly excited and trusting of your body and of birth, you automatically go into your birthing zone.

Midwives often say that women can seem quite spaced out during birth. Many mums who have given birth more than once say that they were in a zone while in labour and not really aware of anything going on around them. Women rarely recall the details of their baby's birth because they were in their birthing zone, which is different to our normal daily levels of awareness.

During labour your brain waves slow down. You may experience this as something similar to feeling sleepy, daydreaming, being in hypnosis or using a mindful meditation. Both hypnosis and mindfulness work so well alongside birth because they help you to stay in your birthing zone, or to get back if anything disturbs you or takes you out of it. They can help if you just feel you need something to keep you centred and focused. You'll learn much more about your birthing zone in Chapter 4.

BENEFITS IN PREGNANCY

If you are preparing for your birth using hypnotherapy, and practising every day, you will experience the positive knock-on effects of being more relaxed, sleeping better and generally feeling more comfortable physically. Women report insomnia lifting and heartburn disappearing once they begin to take the time out to listen to their hypnosis tracks or to meditate.

Unlike many other treatments during pregnancy, hypnotherapy and meditation are non-invasive and can be safely used to help manage certain conditions such as heartburn, sickness and insomnia. They can also be used as simple ways to de-stress, relax and let go, allowing you time to connect with and reflect on your baby.

When you are in a hypnotic or a mindful state, you are deeply relaxed. With hypnotherapy your conscious mind drifts off and any bothersome or troublesome thoughts disappear while you let go, allowing yourself to be guided by someone else's voice that calms you. Being mindful can bring awareness to the moment, of your body and your growing baby. It can be a very rewarding method of connecting with your baby and with physical changes that are occurring within you. The more you get used to being in those states and feeling safe in your surroundings during pregnancy, the more easily you will be able to apply them to the birth.

When you reach this state of deep hypnosis, your muscles relax and your baby often moves in response to these good feelings.

How often does your baby start moving just as you are drifting off to sleep? It's because when you let go mentally, your muscles relax, allowing baby more space to move and stretch. You and your baby will benefit from the time that you take to use mind relaxation techniques.

By using the techniques in this book, you can train yourself to go into self-hypnosis, and to use the simple visualisations to help manage anything that may be troubling or worrying you. Listening to hypnosis tracks is a simple way of accessing the benefits that these techniques have during pregnancy.

WHAT WILL MY MIDWIFE THINK?

Six years ago, you may have got a raised eyebrow if you'd mentioned hypnobirthing to your midwife. Today, thanks to the thousands of people practising and experiencing births using this approach, more and more midwives are witnessing the benefits first hand and welcoming those births. When I am working as a doula – a birth companion – and hypnosis is on the mother's birth plan, I often get midwives who are interested in the approach. I like to think that hospitals match you with a midwife who suits your needs as a couple, and if you have hypnobirthing on your preferences you will get a midwife who is interested in supporting you. If this doesn't happen and you don't feel your midwife is fully supportive, or you feel uncomfortable, it is within your rights to speak to the supervisor of midwives, the midwife in charge of that shift, or request another midwife.

If you have a community midwife you can invite her to share in your preparation. Talk to her about how you would like her to help you and ask her medical questions to help you clarify the choices on your birth plan. If you are having your baby in hospital, make sure that your birth preferences reflect the fact that you are using hypnosis and request that staff help create the right environment (see page 104).

By working with your unconscious, hypnosis preparation will help you to establish a positive connection between your body and your mind during labour. Mindfulness will help you tune in to your instinctive body, allowing you to recognise signals to move your body in a way that will help your baby get into the perfect position for birth. Mindful hypnobirthing will change your negative beliefs about your body and birth at a deep unconscious level, allowing you to be centred and in control.

SUMMARY

- Hypnosis is a way of letting go and relaxing deeply.
- When you are in hypnosis your body will continue to do what it's meant to do.
- Mindfulness is a method to help you stay centred in the present moment.
- When you practise these techniques regularly you will find you sleep better and feel calmly excited about the birth of your baby.

2

THE BENEFITS OF A MINDFUL HYPNOBIRTH

Birth is not only about making babies. Birth is about making mothers — strong, competent, capable mothers who trust themselves and know their inner strength.

Barbara Katz Rothman

Preparing for a mindful hypnobirth brings benefits for you, your partner and your baby. These are different to many other antenatal preparations. You may be surprised to discover that the elements of emotional and mental preparation bring attention to aspects of the birth or parenting which may not have even come into your conscious awareness. It will prepare you in more ways than you can imagine, and when you are emotionally centred and strong you'll be much more in control.

BENEFITS FOR MUM

Birth and Motherhood

Whether the prospect of giving birth excites or frightens you, the closer you get to birth the more you will focus on it, rather than your pregnancy or preparing for the first weeks after your baby is born. After having her first baby, a very good friend of mine asked, 'Why are we so focused on the birth when it is part of so much more and the start of a bigger and more intense journey?' Birth is important, very important, but she's right – it's also vital to recognise the moment of birth as part of a journey, a moment of transition. Baby moves from life inside the womb to life outside the womb, just like a plant that grows under the soil and then breaks the surface, turning towards the sun and growing well as it is nurtured and cared for.

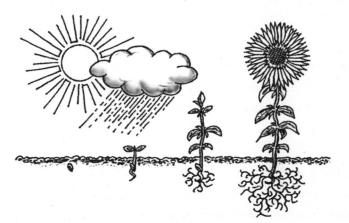

A baby grows like a seed, at first protected and nourished under the ground, then when in sight continuing to grow nourished by the loving care of parents.

During the months you are pregnant your body is growing and expanding. You may be looking forward to your bump showing and being able to feel your baby's movements. You may be following progress through books or online, week by week, being witness to how your baby is changing and growing. How much time have you spent actually thinking about how *your* body changes during pregnancy? How focused are you on those significant changes?

Stop for a moment to reflect on how your body expands to accommodate your baby, building an internal life support system that grows a heart and lungs, tiny feet, eyes and a brain. It's extraordinary and it just does it without you thinking about it. You may be aware of stretching and of tweaks and pressure as your body softens and expands, but accept these as your pregnancy journey.

Fear of pregnancy does exist, but certainly not to the same degree that people are frightened of birth. Some studies show that four in five women are anxious about birth. This means that there is an 80 per cent chance that you have anxieties or worries about birth. Why is this? First of all, many women today don't really understand the physiology of birth; they aren't taught about their bodies nor how incredible the physical changes are that enable our babies to be born. I often hear women say, 'How is that going to get out of there?' without taking the time to learn how the tissues in the body soften and expand for birth, just as they do during pregnancy.

Emotional changes take place too. During your pregnancy you may have a deep sense of knowing that life will change; you may feel that you have little control over how these changes in your life will happen. This can be very unsettling at an unconscious level, though it may not be something you really feel the need to analyse or think about consciously.

The 'thoughts and feelings' element of birth is sometimes sidelined by clinicians. They may separate the physical from the psychological, and see birth as a solely medical event. Yet the physical nature of birth is interwoven with your emotional wellbeing during your birth and in the weeks afterwards.

Embracing Birth as a Transition

Birth is a shift in a journey that started when your baby was conceived, a journey that will go on past birth, into those early years, through to adolescence and adulthood. It's a jumping-off point and a transition, where your relationship with your baby will change. Your baby will no longer be protected within you and the unique relationship you share with your baby while he or she is in your womb will alter. The bond will always be there after your baby is born, but will change and grow.

Women feel this upcoming shift unconsciously. Giving birth is not just bringing your baby into the world; it's also a form of letting go and separation, the first of many that will happen during your child's life. It will happen again at nursery or pre-school, then at primary school, then in a different way when they move on to secondary school and finally leave home. Understanding this and preparing to make that shift is a very important part of birth preparation. The willingness to let go and surrender to the experience of birth is also an acceptance of the shift into motherhood.

From my own experience I knew that there is a need in most women (conscious or unconscious) to experience something sacred when giving birth. From the many women who came to see me, I knew that most wanted to experience the birth of their child as a fulfilling, joyous and creative act. It seemed that all too often, this was denied them, as the psychological and spiritual dimensions of the birth process went largely unacknowledged.

Benig Mauer

The moment of birth is a moment of personal growth and change. Giving life is a powerful experience that can transform you in the deepest parts of your being. Naturally, this can trigger an unconscious sense of sadness or unease. This is especially true of the final stages of birth, just before baby is born. Sometimes I see a mother very tense in these final moments, and I say to her, 'I know you're scared but it's okay to let go. I care about you and I am here for you.' The acknowledgment of her fear with loving support can sometimes be all she needs to hear in that moment. It can enable her to let go and move into the next stage of her journey as a mother.

Birth can teach you how capable you are and how strong you can be. What better preparation could there be for motherhood? In many communities across the world, young men still go through initiation ceremonies into adulthood that test their endurance emotionally and physically, and take them further within themselves than they have gone before. Many people see birth as the female equivalent of this stage in life.

Take a moment to think back on your life and of moments that have helped you grow and become the person you are. Often those moments are ones that may have challenged you; they may have been forced upon you or you may have chosen them. Importantly, they are moments that have moved you forwards, made you stronger and more aware of your own capabilities. This is what birth is, a supremely unique moment in time that you will be able to look back on and say, 'Wow, I did that. What an incredible thing to experience and achieve.'

> *It was the most amazing experience I have ever been through. It took me to a deep place and made me realise who I am and what I am really capable of. I now know that I have spent the last 37 years working at 75 per cent of my true potential but giving birth has allowed me to see what I am truly capable of.*

During birth you may reach a point where you think you can do no more. There may be moments when you doubt yourself and you may ask for help. Others may want to help you, perhaps with drugs, which may distract you or break your rhythm. Drugs may also dampen down the experience of birth and stop you from being able to respond to how your body needs to move or react during labour to help your baby get into the best position for birth. Yet it is this moment when you will be able, if well supported, to push beyond what you know you can do. It is in this moment that you will discover what you are really capable of.

BENEFITS FOR DAD

Getting in Touch with Emotions and Feelings

Your partner may have prepared for his practical role at the birth. For example, he may be ready to get your birth bag in the car, know where the parking is at the hospital, make sure you have things to eat and drink during labour and perhaps how to give you a massage during the birth.

However, just like you, he will also begin preparing emotionally in the months leading up to the birth. He may be aware of the responsibility of providing for a family, of being a father and role model. He may be excited; he may be worried about caring for you during the birth.

The benefits of a mindful hypnobirth are that your partner may feel more emotionally engaged with your pregnancy and the birth of your baby. Taking time to prepare together, sharing your thoughts and fears in a reflective and considered way, can make a real difference to how you prepare for the journey of parenthood together.

Learning the differences between practical preparation and emotional preparation can stand a partner in good stead. If your partner knows how important it is to give you space and to let go of their fears around the birth it can help you tremendously. By addressing these fears during pregnancy you will create a deeper connection that comes from a place of love, not fear, at the birth.

> *Ed's encouragement and support were invaluable in keeping me focused and strong – he really was a peaceful papa. Thinking about his role and preparing him for the big event was totally invaluable!*

A birth can test a partner too and in many ways is an exercise in mindfulness and letting go of judgments.

BENEFITS FOR BABY

A Soothing Life in the Womb

Your baby, so warm and comfortable in their watery world with the muffled sound of your heartbeat to soothe them, will experience a transition themselves. How would you feel descending on an alien planet that had just a few echoes of your home?

Your mindful hypnobirth practice during pregnancy also prepares baby for the birth. Your baby feels your emotions and your environment, so if you are relaxed your baby is relaxed. If there is a loud bang your baby reacts by jumping. When you go to sleep at night and snuggle down into your bed your baby starts moving in response to you letting go of the day's tension.

There is more and more research that explores the impact of what's known as peri-natal psychology, the study of the infant brain and maternal brain before and after birth. Sometimes this research may be alarming for those of us who have suffered from stress or depression during or after pregnancy. Yet it's important for women to know that when you take time out to relax and let go your baby is getting huge benefits. If you have a stressful job, recognise the benefit to your baby of taking time out during each day. Even just five minutes listening to your pregnancy affirmations (the second hypnosis track with this book) can bring real benefits.

From Womb to World

When you go into labour the preparation you have done will help your baby respond well. Imagine your baby in your womb, where they have been for nine months, comfortably listening to your heartbeat and the muffled sounds outside, their eyes closed yet aware of bright light being shone on your belly. Baby has been cushioned from knocks and bumps by your waters. Even as labour starts, each contraction, each tightening or pressure is like a firm massage, slowly and gently palpating and awakening the nerve endings in your baby's arms and legs. In a hypnobirth, you will be calm and relaxed in a loving and supportive environment. Your baby will have a sense of that as well and will benefit from your natural endorphins.

Your baby moves down the birth canal with each contraction and is eventually born into a very different world to the one they know. Very often, even in an undisturbed birth, there will be bright lights and sharp noises, rather than the darkness and muffled sounds they are used to. Baby may be taken away from their mother, rubbed down with a towel and put on a cold hard set of scales. Any sense of familiarity is gone in that instant. Only your voice, your partner's voice and your smell are familiar anchors in that new and foreign place.

Making sure that your baby's transition into the world is as gentle and tranquil as possible can settle and calm them. Often babies born into calmer environments don't cry as much, if at all, after the birth. As mothers, we can take responsibility to minimise intervention as much as possible by being informed but also by being more trusting in our bodies, taking responsibility for our births and being mindful of our choices.

Keeping your birth as stress free as possible, for yourself and for your baby, is important. You can do that by focusing on how your state of mind impacts upon your decisions, your experiences and your physical wellbeing during labour. Even if your birth takes a different course than expected, being able to stay calm and focused has a positive impact on your baby. In prolonged states of anxiety during labour, the oxygen supply to your baby is reduced. If you are anxious and your heart is beating fast, research shows your baby's is too; if you are relaxed, centred and calm your baby will benefit. I regularly get comments from midwives that when mum is calm and in a good state of mind, it's reflected in how well baby responds to labour. Your baby will benefit from you being centred and confident, giving birth from a place not of fear but of strength.

SUMMARY

- The benefits of a mindful hypnobirth are not just for you but for your partner and your baby as well.
- The benefits can last long after the birth and can have a genuinely positive impact on you, your baby and your partner.
- A mindful hypnobirth allows you to connect with your body and create a calm emotional and physical environment.
- Your preparation will help you birth your baby not from a place of fear but from a place of love, trust and strength.

3

GETTING READY FOR A MINDFUL HYPNOBIRTH

Our willingness to embody new beginnings mirrors the biggest new beginning of all. After all the preparation and hard work the child is born, and with it, the mother.

Jon Kabat-Zinn

Hypnobirthing is a commitment. When you choose to prepare using mindful hypnobirthing, you need to do more than just read the book and the techniques once. You will need to find time to learn to use these techniques until your body masters them without you even having to think about it. This is called conditioning, and conditioning is a learned response; when you learn to do something, the more you do it, the more your body reacts without your mind getting involved.

GETTING YOUR BIRTH BRAIN INTO CONDITION

Conditioning was famously discovered in an experiment called Pavlov's dogs. The physiologist Ivan Pavlov wanted to learn more about learned and automatic behaviour. In this experiment, whenever Pavlov gave food to his dogs, he also rang a bell. After a short while, just ringing the bell would cause the dogs to salivate. This helped psychologists to understand that a learned association could create an automatic physical response in the body.

Milton Erikson, a famous hypnotherapist, used what he called the lemon sherbert experiment to demonstrate conditioning and association. You can try this now. Either read it first and then follow the exercise or ask your partner or a friend to read it to you while you have your eyes closed. If you don't like lemon, substitute it with something you do enjoy eating.

> Close your eyes and imagine that you have a lemon sherbert in your hand. Be aware of the weight and the pressure of the lemon sherbert in the palm of your hand. Look at the lemon sherbert, imagine how that lemon sherbert is going to taste. Then with your other hand imagine taking the lemon sherbert and putting it in your mouth. Be aware of the sharpness of the lemon flavour as you turn the lemon sherbert over in your mouth. Switch the lemon sherbert from one side of your mouth to the other and then either let it dissolve or crunch it, aware of the feeling and flavours in your mouth.

You may be aware of your mouth starting to produce saliva. You may also have pursed your lips as you imagined the tartness of the lemon. Your body is responding to that suggestion of the lemon sherbert in your mouth even though it's not really there. What your preparation will do is teach your body, through conditioning, to automatically respond to certain suggestions, thoughts, feelings, surroundings and people in a positive and relaxed way during labour.

PRACTICE MAKES PERFECT

You must find time every day to practise the techniques you learn. Women who really benefit from the techniques have been dedicated in listening to their hypnosis tracks and practising their exercises, both with and without their partners. As you become familiar with the techniques you will learn in the book, you will feel more and more confident. Not only will you be able to use them to help you stay calm and focused, but you will also be confident enough to adapt and change them in a way that is perfect for you. The image of the baby surfing on page 85 is from a mother who came to my class; she had really made the techniques her own and had the image of a surfing baby on the wall throughout her labour.

Hypnosis is able to harness your own beliefs and thoughts, using them in a way to change how you feel and react. I don't know what your personal thoughts and feelings are about birth, but I do know that the techniques in this book are expplained in a way that will enable you to adapt and change them for your own benefit so that they are consistent with the type of birth you are planning. Regular practice will help you do that. As you practise, other images and symbols or methods may come into your awareness; if so, use them.

Practise with your birth partner if you can. It will help you condition yourself to their voice and touch, and they will become more confident in using the techniques. If your partner works away, see if a friend can help you. Setting time aside with your partner at least once a week can be a great way of preparing together and can help your partner become more mindfully aware of your pregnancy and your baby.

How to Set up a Practice Space

To practise the techniques in this book, find a space where you won't be disturbed. Many women like to do one of the mindfulness or hypnosis exercises just before going to bed. This is a great option as you are less likely to be disturbed, and the side-effect of the hypnosis tracks is great sleep!

As you get used to practising, it can be helpful to try it out in different spaces and test yourself in noisier locations. You'll find that you are increasingly able to let go of sounds and noises, and much more adept at turning your attention inwards and switching off. You can listen to the exercises while travelling to work by train, in a quiet room at work or, if you have other children, while they are having a nap. Some women also like to practise in the bath or outside in the fresh air. Anywhere is fine as long as you feel safe, secure and comfortable. Practising at different times of the day and in noisier places means that you are learning how to drift in and out of hypnosis easily and quickly. Perfect preparation for labour.

Practice Positions

You can practise in lots of different positions. Although it can be very comfortable lying down on your left side when you listen to your tracks, you don't have to be lying down all the time. The illustrations below show some good positions in which to practise your relaxation or hypnosis techniques. These positions are all beneficial for helping to get your baby into a good position for labour and will feel very comfortable. All the positions you practise in are very good upright positions for labour too.

If you are doing yoga as a form of preparation as well, you can do some of the exercises in simple yoga positions that feel comfortable. Try this for the light relaxation techniques and visualisations or while listening to the hypnosis tracks. The birth preparation track is 30 minutes long, so just be aware that you would have to hold that position for 30 minutes. It may be better for you to listen to the pregnancy or birth affirmations in a yoga pose as they are much shorter.

Think about getting into the sitting positions as much as possible in your day-to-day life, while either at home or at work. Don't underestimate the importance of keeping a good posture during pregnancy. When you are in good positions it helps your baby get into position. If your baby is in a good position it can make labour a lot quicker and easier. Be especially mindful of your position when you are relaxing as when your abdominal muscles relax, baby often moves more. Avoid slouching, particularly during mindful hypnobirthing practice.

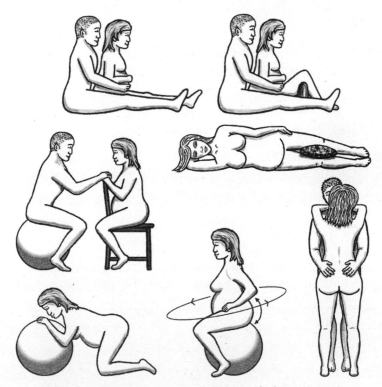

These positions can be used for listening to the hypnosis tracks, practising your breathing and also during labour.

> **TIP:** Get yourself a teacup and a teaspoon. Put the teaspoon head down in the teacup. Now, holding the teacup in your hand, slouch into your sofa. You'll notice that the handle of the teaspoon slides to the back of the teacup. If you sit upright and tilt your pelvis forward, the handle of the teacup swings around to the front. Imagine your baby's spine is the handle of the spoon and the teacup is your body. This is a great visual guide to helping you think about your position.

SETTING YOUR BIRTH INTENTION

Hypnosis is about focus and direction but you have to know where you are going, otherwise you can get sidetracked. With clients who are working towards certain feelings they wish to experience, I always make sure that they have set a goal and then work towards that goal. To set your course, you must set your goal and decide how you want to experience your birth.

What is important for you? You may want to be more in control; you may want to be more confident; you may want to be calm; you may want to comfortably let go. The techniques that you practise will create strong roots to help you stay focused and centred during labour.

Imagine that you are a tree moving in the wind. The wind may turn into a gale or it may be a gentle breeze, but because you are well prepared your roots are strong and you are able to bend and sway. The techniques are your roots but they have to be nurtured; you do this through careful preparation. Instead of being blown about, afraid of being uprooted, you are able to stay rooted and calm with a deep conviction that you are strong, centred and safe.

You will find your tree, just like the one below, at www. mindful-hypnobirthing.co.uk. Print off your tree, and fill the branches up with elements that you sense are important to you at the birth. Stick it up somewhere that you will see often, maybe in your bedroom or in your kitchen.

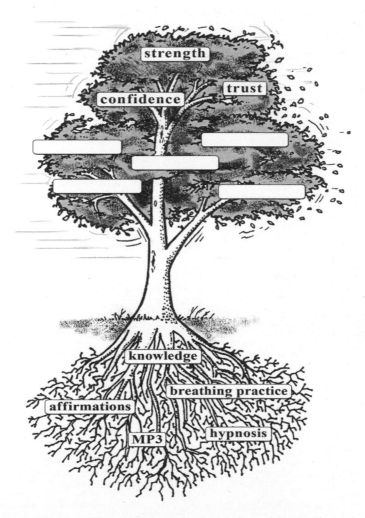

Imagine your tree, and reflect on how you wish to approach your birth emotionally. Recognise that the practice you put in during pregnancy builds strong and sturdy roots that help keep you grounded and centred.

LISTENING TO YOUR HYPNOSIS TRACKS

You'll find that you have three hypnosis tracks to download with this book at www.mindful-hypnobirthing.co.uk:

- Birth preparation (30 minutes)
- Pregnancy affirmations (5 minutes)
- Birth affirmations (5 minutes)

Listen to the birth preparation, pregnancy affirmations and birth affirmations at least three times a week up to weeks 28–32. You may want to listen to them every day all the way through as I did when I was pregnant. For me, it was time to switch off from my job and any stresses in my life, and it helped me sleep so well – don't forget that these are some of the real benefits of practice to be gained during pregnancy.

After around 28–32 weeks, you will be in a deeper part of you. Perhaps out of your direct awareness you may be preparing more for the birth. You may experience a shift in how you are feeling that you are unable to put into words, or perhaps you may actively start to reflect more on the birth ahead. At this point you should switch to using all three tracks every day if you can. Playing them back-to-back for a 40-minute relaxation session is fine. The hypnosis tracks are filled with suggestions that help form those strong roots in your tree, and which build your unconscious belief and trust in the process of birth.

Do not listen to the hypnosis tracks while driving or operating machinery. Once you've listened to them a few times you'll know why! You may feel like you are falling asleep; that's fine. Hypnosis sometimes feels like that but it's just your thinking brain switching off. Even if you do fall asleep, your unconscious mind will still be absorbing messages, so enjoy the rest if you do. Rest assured that people will always wake up and come back into the room when they want to, no matter how deeply in hypnosis they are.

If you can, listen to the hypnosis tracks with stereo headphones as they use a specific hypnosis technique called dual induction, which really benefits from stereo headphones.

Practice Guidelines

While a lot of women like to go with the flow, many also find it helpful to have a timetable set out. Having a goal every day can be very helpful in keeping you going in your practice. When you are busy at work and have a lot on in your life it can be easy to say, 'I'll do it tomorrow.' Having a guide will help you stick to your mindful hypnobirth plan.

Practise your breathing, 'three, two, one, relax, relax, relax' (see page 46) and hypnosis deepener (see page 48)	Every day for 15 minutes
Listen to your MP3	At least three times a week up to week 32 and then every day
Read your affirmations	Every day
Practise with your partner	At least once a week
Watch a great birth video	Once a week
Read a book from the Books sections at the back of this book	At your own pace

SUMMARY

- Hypnosis is all about conditioning, repetition and association.
- Mindfulness is about becoming familiar with the rhythms of your body.
- Practising over and over again will mean that your body will respond while your brain can stay calm, focused and relaxed in your birthing zone.
- Set your goal; find a place and a time to get started on your mindful hypnobirthing journey.

4

GETTING TO KNOW YOUR BIRTHING ZONE

A woman is the full circle. Within her is the power to create, nurture and transform.

Diane Mariechild

Earlier, I briefly mentioned your birthing zone, the place where your mind should be when you are birthing (see page 16). When you are in your birthing zone your brain waves slow down. It's a familiar state to everyone, and is similar to that moment of not quite being awake and not quite being asleep. Many mums don't remember all the details of their births because they were deep within their birthing zone. In your birthing zone you lose track of time and turn awareness to what's happening internally rather than externally. The human part of you stops getting in the way by thinking about doing it and lets the animal part of you just do it, as it's done for thousands of years for your ancestors.

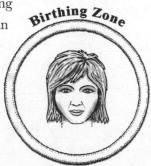

Many women naturally go into this state during birth and this may be the same for you. Other women may need techniques to help them stay in their zone, particularly if something takes them out of that zone. This could be a loud noise, an interruption or a change of scenery. Hypnosis and mindfulness exercises, as well as love and support, will help keep you in – or help you get back into – your birthing zone.

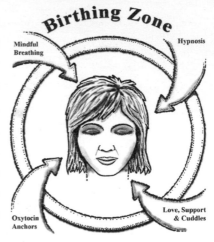

When you go into your birthing zone, you are quietening down the part of your brain that is alert and chatty. I like to call this part of the brain the chattering chimp; it's the part that is constantly wondering and asking why, how and what. When you slow this part of your brain down you rely on automatic responses from your old brain, the part of your brain that knows how to birth, just as all other mammals know how to birth.

ARE YOU AN ANIMAL OR A HUMAN?

Humans are mammals and physically there is little difference in how we and other mammals respond to our hormones during labour. I watched a programme showing a giraffe giving birth. The zookeeper, standing well back from the giraffe's pen, whispers furtively to the cameraman, 'Stand back a bit, lights off, she mustn't know we are here.' Then the giraffe is shown swaying and moving around her pen, even getting down on to her front haunches; her calf just slips out and she nudges herself up. The zookeeper is the perfect midwife; he understands that if she knew they were there it might disturb her and affect the birth. He knows that interrupting her after the birth will affect bonding with her calf.

This demonstrates that the giraffe wasn't taught what to do; she knew what to do. She had no birth manuals telling her how to birth her calf or what to expect, nor did she have someone directing her course of labour. So why is it so much harder for us as humans?

THE CHATTERING CHIMP

I've already mentioned the chattering chimp, also referred to as the monkey mind, which is the part of our brain that is more complex than that of other mammals. The Buddha likened our mind to a monkey: 'Just as a monkey, swinging through a forest wilderness, grabs a branch. Letting go of it, it grabs another branch. Letting go of that, it grabs another one. Letting go of that, it grabs another one. In the same way, what's called "mind", "intellect", or "consciousness" by day and by night arises as one thing and ceases as another.' The part of our brain that behaves in this way is known as the neo-cortex, or the new brain. It is responsible for many things, but it's the aspects of reasoning, self-awareness, conscious thought and language that have the biggest impact on how we experience birth.

We need to reduce activity in our neo-cortex during labour. It's the part we switch off when we go to sleep or use meditation and hypnosis, which is why the techniques you will learn work so well. In hypnosis we often talk about this as 'bypassing the critical mind'. Your birthing zone is in your old brain. When your neo-cortex becomes still and quiet, it allows the instinctive animal – the lioness within – to awaken. This is the part that knows how to birth.

How Thinking Gets in the Way of a Great Birth

Self-awareness sits in our neo-cortex, and can be very problematic when it comes to birth. Birth is a naturally primal event. It's related to instinctive responses connected to reproduction, release of bodily fluids and so on, yet as humans we are trained to do these privately.

Our new brain, along with cultural and social conditioning, can sometimes get in the way of birth by saying, 'Stop! You can't do this in front of him/her.'

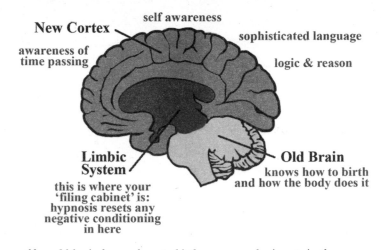

Your old brain knows how to birth, your new brain gets in the way.

Second-time mothers who come and talk to my class are very reassuring to first-time mothers. One in particular made me laugh. She said to the class that her biggest fear during the birth was pooing in front of her husband and the midwife. She made a big joke of it and said that when it happened it really didn't matter; in fact she didn't even notice. It's true to say that many second-time mothers lose the inhibitions that first-time mothers sometimes have. They also just know that they can do it. A birth story I once received said, 'I did not even realise I was at the pushing phase until her head appeared – my body really must have taken over.' When you know this it's easy to let go and shut your chattering chimp down. There is nothing to discuss; you accept, embrace and allow your contractions and your body to do their job. I believe that many second-time mums have easier births partly because of this.

A paramedic once told me a story of a woman who had been pregnant when she was admitted to an intensive care unit. Although she was in a coma, she gave birth with no difficulty at around eight months. In fact, the nurses only noticed as the head was emerging. Because her neo-cortex was resting, her body could birth her baby completely uninterrupted by thoughts.

Another activity that our new brain does is analyse. We take information from the past, from what we have already learned, and apply it to what may happen in the future. We do this by applying any number of possibilities to the present, which can influence how we act in that moment and the choices we make. When it comes to birth this is a really disabling factor for humans and gets in the way. Other mammals have the advantage that their body gets on and does it without them thinking 'Is that normal?', 'What does that mean?', 'Will what happened to my friend Alice happen to me?' Later on we'll go into more detail about why these thoughts can slow labour down or stop it altogether (see page 56).

DISCOVERING YOUR BIRTHING ZONE

When we go to sleep, our chattering chimp sleeps too. I want you to close your eyes and think about what you need in your room when you go to sleep at night. Make a list. It may need to be dark, tidy, quiet; you may like it warm or cool. Your doors will be secure, curtains or blinds probably closed. This is the type of environment in which your chattering chimp likes to rest. You may find that if you are thinking a lot and have something on your mind it's harder to silence that chattering chimp and go to sleep.

With the techniques you are learning you are training your neo-cortex to quieten down. You are discovering how to lull your chattering chimp to sleep and to rest while you get into your birthing zone and your body instinctively births your baby.

Staying in your Birthing Zone

There are three simple steps to staying in your birthing zone and keeping that chattering chimp at bay. These are the foundations for every visualisation or other hypnosis technique in this book. You'll need to learn to be mindfully present in your birthing zone to allow yourself to stay in touch with your body, centred and strong.

The first step is tuning into the rhythm of your breath and creating your birth mantra. You may find that staying mindfully with your breath is as much as you need; often women say that when they have regularly practised this it is very easy to stay rooted in the birthing zone. Step two takes you deeper into relaxation and triggers your muscles to relax. As you get to step three you enter a much deeper state of hypnosis, shutting out external disturbances and turning your focus within.

Before doing any of the visualisations or other exercises in the book, follow the first three steps detailed below. You should practise these techniques every day for at least 10 minutes, in addition to listening to your hypnosis tracks. Find somewhere quiet and have the Mindful Hypnobirth instrumental hypnosis track on quietly in the background. It can be helpful to set a timer for five minutes. Then, as you get used to practising it and feel that the timer is going off too soon, train yourself to stretch the time out to 10 minutes, 15 minutes and even longer if you wish.

Step 1: Mindful Breathing

You breathe every day without thinking, but how often do you sit quietly and pay attention to your breath? When you turn attention to your breathing, in pregnancy or during labour, your focus turns inwards and shifts away from other things in your environment that might unsettle you or take you out of your birthing zone. At first, some people find it difficult to stop their mind wandering, and say, 'I can't stop thinking about other things.' Mindfulness is called a practice: the more you do it the easier it becomes. You'll find that you will be able to find a stillness that really helps you connect with your body and your baby without the clutter of life getting in the way.

When you are focused on something like your breath, your brain is unable to focus on something else. Your conscious mind is only able to hold a very small amount of information at any one time. This is a great skill to have when giving birth. Being able to use your breath to keep you in your birthing zone is a simple and effective technique.

1. To start you need to ensure that you are taking deep abdominal breaths. Put one hand on your chest and one hand on your belly. Close your eyes and become aware of which hand is moving more than the other. If the hand on your chest is moving, you need to take deeper breaths so your belly feels as if it's breathing in and out and the hand on your belly is moving more.

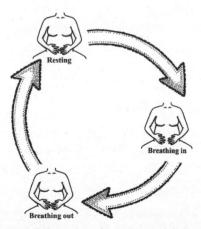

Put this up in your home somewhere, or at work, and stop regularly to practise this rhythm every now and again for just a few minutes.

2. Follow that breath, breathing in to a count of six and out to eight. When your out-breath is longer than your in-breath this is called a 'lengthening breath'. If you have been doing pregnancy yoga you may know this better as the golden thread. Alternatively, you may prefer just breathing slowly in and slowly out, aware of the warmth of the air as you breathe and your breath moving down through your body and out again. What's most important when practising your birth breath is that you get into a comfortable and familiar rhythm. You'll find at the end of the out-breath that you will automatically rest for between one and three seconds before taking another breath.

3. When you are learning to quieten your mind, following your breath, you may find that you get caught up in everyday thoughts and feelings. This is normal when you start practising. Every time you find yourself doing this, bring yourself back to your breathing and say in your mind, 'Breathing in and breathing out.' Free yourself of any judgments that say you can't do it because you can; it just takes daily practice.

> **TIP:** You can also add a mantra to this to help keep you centred, especially if you find your thoughts wandering a lot. 'I breathe in I am strong; I breathe out I let go.' 'I breathe in, in this moment I can do this; I breathe out I relax.'

Step 2: Light Muscle Relaxation

Once you have settled into your breathing and have a comfortable rhythm, breathing in and breathing out, you can start to allow your muscles to relax even more. This light hypnosis exercise is called 'Three, two, one, relax, relax, relax'. You can condition your body to respond to this command so that your muscles let go and relax quickly and easily. This is a great technique and can be used for all sorts of events in life such as giving a presentation, playing sports or before an exam.

Once you have mastered it you can apply it to anything you want for the rest of your life. A woman I once knew had learned the same thing in a slightly different way for the birth of her daughter in the 1960s and said she still benefited from it in her everyday life years later. Whenever she felt anxious or a bit stressed, or before a big event, she used her breathing and her muscle relaxation to centre herself. It's important to trust that this will happen, even if you think it hasn't worked or you aren't aware of your muscles relaxing. A friend regularly uses this technique when she plays tennis; if she's cross or uptight over a bad serve, she says, 'Three, two, one, relax, relax, relax,' and even if she can't feel the inhibiting tension disappear, she knows it has because she always hits a great serve afterwards.

Imagine that you are somewhere outside where you feel very comfortable, happy and warm. Become aware of the warmth of the sun on your head, making your hair feel warm.

3. Allow that warmth to travel down your body through your head and chest …
2. through your abdomen and pelvis, allowing that area to relax deeply …
1. now down through your calves and ankles to your feet and toes.

Then say relax, relax, relax.
Each time you say, 'Three, two, one, relax, relax, relax,' your muscles will let go of any tension. This will help you centre yourself and tune in to your body.

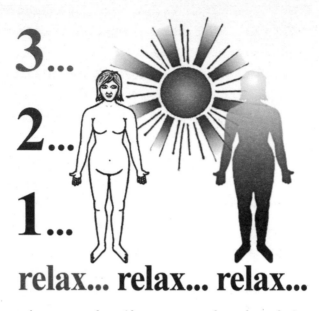

3...
2...
1...
relax... relax... relax...

As you count down 'three, two, one, relax, relax, relax',
all the muscles in your body will let go, your jaw and hands
will relax and your shoulders will release any tension.

> **TIP:** You can put this image up in your home somewhere where you can see it all the time. Just looking at it will embed that sense of relaxation with the counting down so that your muscles respond, unconsciously relaxing.

Step 3: Hypnosis Deepener

A hypnosis deepener is a way of taking someone into a deeper state of hypnosis. You're going to learn it in a very simple way that you can either do yourself, or your partner can learn to do with you. After you've established the rhythm of your breath and have done 'Three, two, one, relax, relax, relax', count down from 10 to 1, slowly in your head.

Make yourself comfortable and focus on your breathing. Get a regular breath and, when you feel your shoulders soften and begin to sink into your body, say, 'Three, two, one, relax, relax, relax.' Your shoulders will soften even more. Now close your eyes and slowly count back in your head: 10, 9, 8, 7, 6, 5, 4, 3, 2, 1. Imagine a place where you feel very comfortable and secure. It may be a place in your home or it may be outside, but it's somewhere that you feel relaxed. Just allow yourself to spend as much time imagining yourself there as you can, and open your eyes when you are done.

TIP: Your partner can do this with you, reading out the description above in a slow, soft voice. As they count, ask them to include something positive between each number. For example, 10 you're doing really well … 9 that's perfect … 8 follow your breath … just let go … 7 I am here for you … 6 that's brilliant … 5 all your muscles relaxed now … 4 doing great … 3 perfect … 2 follow your breath … breathe in and breathe out … 1 very comfortable, centred and strong. You can stretch this out by counting down from 20 if you wish.

SUMMARY

- Get used to being in your birthing zone with steps 1, 2 and 3.
- Learn to quieten your mind with the rhythm of your breath.
- Practise the hypnosis deepener with your birth partner.

5

LETTING GO OF FEAR AND ANXIETY

Giving birth should be your greatest achievement, not your greatest fear.

Jane Weideman

Your body and your mind are intrinsically connected when it comes to birth. Your own life experiences and beliefs, from the moment you are born up until the present day, can trigger automatic physical responses in your body, sometimes overpowering what you consciously want to experience.

In this chapter I'm going to tell you much more about why fear and expectation of pain may create pain. Understanding how your brain can get in the way of a good birth experience will help you to recognise and release your fears around birth. That way you create the space within you to allow your body to birth freely without tension and anxiety that fear can create. At the end of this chapter you'll have addressed and let go of any fears, preparing yourself for setting new positive beliefs around birth in Chapter 6.

YOUR BODY: THE PERFECT MACHINE

Do you really understand how your body works during labour? Most teenage girls receive very limited sex education and grow up unfamiliar with their body and what happens to it during birth.

Have you stopped to think about how your body is growing a complex human being from an egg and a sperm? Over the nine months you are pregnant your body will construct a heart, lungs, eyes and kidneys, without your brain even thinking about it. That's incredible. Scientists have spent years trying to construct organs artificially but you have done it without even thinking.

Your fist-sized womb will expand to accommodate your growing baby and their little world. The body will undergo enormous changes during pregnancy but women tend to accept these without them becoming a source of anxiety. As your internal organs relocate, with your heart and lungs moving higher to make room for your growing baby, you may get niggles and tweaks. You may have a trapped nerve here and there; maybe a bit of backache or signs that your ligaments are softening.

So while you may accept that your tissues expand and soften to accommodate a baby during pregnancy, what do you think of birth? Do you believe your body can do it? Are you worried about how 'that is going to get out of there', as many women say in my classes? If you think like that, remember it's not a failing of your body but a failure of others to teach you about birth anatomy. Just as your body is designed to support and grow a human baby, your body is designed to birth your baby – in a way that is perfect for you both. Evolution would be deeply flawed if women could grow babies but not birth them. The problem is that when you are frightened of birth, whatever your fear is, it creates changes in your body that can slow labour down, make it more painful and difficult, sometimes stopping it altogether.

HELPFUL HORMONES

To understand how fear affects your body, you first have to understand the role of your hormones in stopping and starting labour. Your hormones are the most sensitive part of your birthing body and how you think, both consciously and unconsciously, interacts with these hormones and can either slow labour down or speed it up.

Let's just say that you think that birth is a normal everyday event. You've been raised in a society that celebrates birth, a society where women are supported and cared for with love during birth and women look forward to birthing their babies. Because of this support and understanding you allow your body to soften and expand in birth just as it does during pregnancy, with full confidence and trust in your body. When this happens your body releases plenty of the birth hormone, known as oxytocin.

Oxytocin

Oxytocin is a bonding hormone – it is the glue that holds our communities together. We are a vulnerable species: on our own we would not survive long in the wild from more powerful predators, so being together in groups and communities keeps us safe and protects us. Even today, research shows that being part of a community, feeling loved and connected, reduces the risk of some illnesses such as heart disease. This sense of community and connection is set within your limbic brain, the old part of your brain. It is based on your experience in the womb, at birth and in your early years through identifying relationships with your parents and those around you.

Oxytocin also helps us nurture our young. Mostly, we produce only one child at a time. We have to look after them properly through nurturing love so they survive and thrive. This is a distinct evolutionary strategy that makes mammals different from other animals and is enhanced by the hormone oxytocin.

Also known as the love hormone, oxytocin encourages reproduction by making sex fun. It also promotes the willingness to give birth. Women who are uninhibited by fear have free-flowing oxytocin during birth. Their birth experiences are often much more positive and self-affirming than many you see on television today.

Beta-endorphins

The undisturbed release of oxytocin then releases beta-endorphins. These are your body's own natural painkillers and feel-good hormones. They can be produced only by naturally occurring oxytocin, not artificial oxytocin.

Beta-endorphins are a gift of nature enabling women to have an incredibly powerful and euphoric birth experience. I've met many women who have said that they want to do it again and again; this is how birth should be. I'm not talking about a pain-free birth, I'm talking about a birth free of suffering and full of power. There is a very subtle difference.

Your Baby Was Born to Be Loved by you

The bonding characteristic of oxytocin also means that your baby is born to be loved and cared for by you. We give birth to our babies very early in their development and they are dependent on their mother for survival. The rush of oxytocin *is* the rush of love we feel for our babies when they are born and bonds us to our babies. Your love for your baby will be their protection.

The benefits of oxytocin are that it:

- lowers your pulse rate and blood pressure
- reduces any sensation of pain in your body
- can dilate blood vessels and create warmth

- accelerates growth and the healing of wounds
- stimulates the release of prolactin for milk production
- supports attachment between you and your baby
- triggers positive responses in the father who bonds with his baby with an equivalent rush of euphoria

'Private Hormone'

Sometimes oxytocin is called the shy hormone, or our private hormone. In order to release oxytocin, you need to feel safe and private. Sarah Buckley, a doctor who specialises in birth hormones, says that the most important message a woman needs to have about birth is that she should feel 'private, safe and unobserved'. This can also mean having someone present but not necessarily staring intently at you. Knitting used to be a very popular task for midwives during a birth. The sound of needles was a soothing reminder from the midwife that 'I am here for you but not watching you'. In some areas of the UK they are reintroducing this skill.

Desmond Morris, a well-known zoologist, observed humans and other mammals giving birth and found similarities. He wrote:

Nine out of ten foals are born in the middle of the night. This is no accident; this is the result of the mares controlling the timing of their contractions. They wait and wait, until they are alone and all is quiet. Only then will they give birth. This is not something they learn. It is an instinctive ability and it helps the mother to make one of her most vulnerable moments also one of her most private.

Adrenaline and Stress Hormones

Adrenaline and nor-adrenaline, on the other hand, are much less welcome visitors during the early stages of labour. Adrenaline and nor-adrenaline are fight, flight or freeze hormones – stress hormones – meaning that when you feel threatened, worried or think you are in danger of being hurt your body activates your sympathetic nervous system to help you get out of danger quickly.

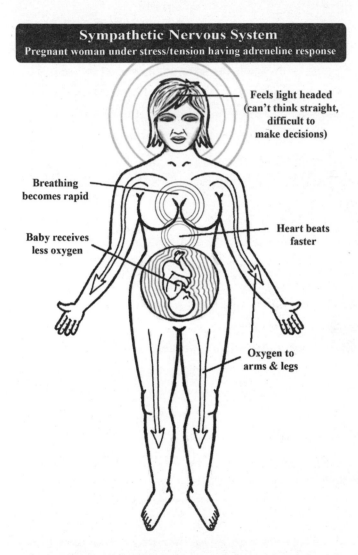

Sympathetic Nervous System
Pregnant woman under stress/tension having adreneline response

Feels light headed (can't think straight, difficult to make decisions)

Breathing becomes rapid

Baby receives less oxygen

Heart beats faster

Oxygen to arms & legs

When you are anxious and afraid, either consciously or unconsciously, your body goes into survival mode and triggers the sympathetic nervous system, known as fight, flight or freeze.

Your blood rushes to your arms and legs so that you can fight or run away. Freezing is also a common response that animals do when they are threatened; it's simply playing dead when there is nowhere to run. It's a safety mechanism.

Adrenaline and nor-adrenaline play an active and normal part of the final moments of labour and a crucial role in helping baby prepare physically for life outside the womb (see page 186). However, it's important to understand how too much adrenaline or nor-adrenaline, too soon in labour, can slow labour down and stop your body doing what it's supposed to do.

HOW FEAR CAN SLOW DOWN BIRTH

Four out of five women have some anxiety about childbirth. Who wouldn't be apprehensive with a 'grit your teeth and get on with it' attitude? Why wouldn't you be frightened if you are constantly told that birth is 'the worst pain you'll ever have', 'just take every drug offered' and 'the only reason we do it again is because we are designed to forget the pain'.

It is true, birth is intense and powerful, and it can feel overwhelming, but it is not considered to be painful by all women who birth. Some women enjoy it and find it much easier than they were led to believe. Some women even have what's known as an orgasmic birth – remember oxytocin is the sex hormone, and when your body is flooded with oxytocin it is primed for what is called an 'ecstatic experience'.

Stay with me! I know about orgasmic birth and I've seen films showing it, but I was as surprised as the eight other couples in one of my classes when one of the mums was forthcoming about her first birth, which she had in hospital and described as orgasmic. She said she would never speak up about it in a toddler group, or to other mums, as it didn't seem right when they were talking about traumatic births. Her experience in hospital had surprised her but she certainly reinforced to the class the value of oxytocin and its feel-good properties during labour.

In a birth that is completely free of fear and when you feel secure and private, oxytocin should flow freely. With each contraction your body sends a message to your brain to produce more oxytocin, and with more oxytocin your body produces more contractions. This is called a positive feedback loop. It's like a private, whispered conversation between your brain and your womb, which gives direction to your body. This loop of conversation helps you to release all the hormones needed for your contractions to happen and for labour to progress.

Fear and anxiety do the exact opposite – they trigger adrenaline and nor-adrenaline, which can slow labour down. Oxytocin and adrenaline are known as antagonists; you can't have them both together. It's like a seesaw effect. The more oxytocin you have the less adrenaline; and the more adrenaline the less oxytocin. As oxytocin goes down, the messages to the womb slow down, which can slow contractions down.

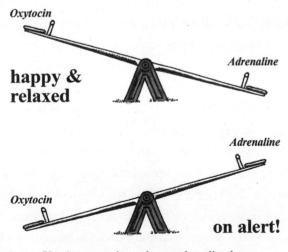

Keeping oxytocin up keeps adrenaline low.

EXPECTATION, ANXIETY, FEAR AND PAIN

Expectation of pain does two things that change our experience of birth. First, expectation can create fear, which in turn triggers the release of adrenaline and tension in your body. Second, it's the expectation of a painful sensation that can create a painful sensation.

In some hypnobirthing programmes, you are not supposed to talk about pain, simply because talking about pain is a suggestion that turns our attention to it. For example, if I said, 'Don't look or think about that plant in the corner of the room,' you immediately become aware of that plant; in fact you can't stop looking at it. You may have many new thoughts associated with that plant. Similarly, with pain and labour, if the suggestion is that there is pain, when we turn our focus to pain we may begin to create an expectation and a very real experience of pain.

Pain is something that fascinates scientists because it is so closely associated with experience and expectation. If we are told to expect pain, we experience pain, even if there is none. Numerous studies in the last 20 years have shown that anxiety of pain increases both pain sensations and unpleasantness of pain. One of the most interesting is a 2011 study by Professor Irene Tracey at Oxford University which showed how our expectation of pain can cause more pain, even overpowering potent painkillers. Tracey's team applied heat to the legs of 22 patients, who were asked to report the level of pain on a scale of 1 to 100. Those patients were attached to an intravenous drip so drugs could be administered secretly. The initial average pain rating was 66. Patients were then given a potent painkiller, without their knowledge, and the pain score went down to 55. They were then told they were being given a painkiller and the score went down to 39. Then, without changing the dose, the patients were told the painkiller had been withdrawn and to expect pain. The score went up to 64, close to the original measure of pain, despite the fact that the potent painkiller was still being administered. The study was corroborated by magnetic resonance imaging, which highlighted which parts of the brain were functioning during the experiment.

Helen was walking down the street when someone looked at her ankle in horror, turned to Helen and said, 'Oh my goodness, you've hurt your ankle really badly. How did you do that?' Helen looked down and saw blood congealing and trickling down her ankle and her foot. She started crying and saying how much it hurt, finding a bench nearby to sit down on. On closer inspection it turned out that the blood was in fact tomato ketchup. It stopped hurting instantly and Helen felt a bit of an idiot. The truth is her brain was expecting the pain and created that feeling. The pain was real to her even though there was no source of that pain.

You may be afraid because of the expectation of pain; pain that other people have told you about. This may create anxiety about how you will cope, as well as labelling the unique sensations of birth as painful. When you do go into labour and your body responds to those unfamiliar sensations, your brain goes through a rapid calculation based on what you know and have been told. If you have been told it is pain, your brain will calculate labour + unfamiliar strong sensation = intense pain. The presence of pain indicates fear that something is wrong and creates tension and anxiety, which can make the pain worse.

Tension and Pain

When we are anxious or afraid our bodies create tension, and tension creates pain. This is commonly referred to as the 'Fear

Tension Pain Cycle'. The research carried out by Irene Tracey's team of neuroscientists shows that people who are anxious are more sensitive to pain, both chronic and temporary.

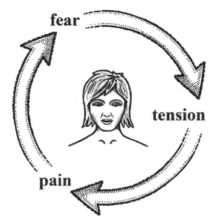

When you are anxious and afraid, tension and pain are more pronounced.

If you have lower levels of anxiety your body will have much more capacity to deal with any physical sensations, and any pain you have will be much less. For some women, birth can be completely painless.

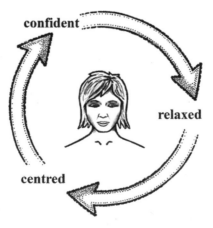

When you are confidently trusting your body, your muscles relax and you experience much more comfortable contractions.

People who have had what they call a pain-free experience of birth describe it not as pain but as a strong, intense sensation. Many second-time mums come to my class because they know they can manage birth and want techniques to help them focus. I strongly believe that a lot of second births are quicker not just because the mother's body has had a baby before, but also because the mum knows deep down that she can do it and what it will be like. A first-time mum may hold the anxiety of all the stories she's been told and a sense of the unknown, creating tension and apprehension as she approaches the birth of her baby.

What Creates Fear?

Fear can be many things: it may be about the physical changes during labour; it may be about the pain that other women have described; it may be about the hospital and procedures themselves. It may even be small anxieties about whether you are going to get to the hospital on time or have got childcare for other children, or whether your husband will get back if he works a distance away.

There may be constant suggestions that things could go wrong and that you may be putting your baby at risk. During pregnancy, your visits to the midwife are made up of tests and checks on the baby. Some of these are vital but others may instil fear where there should be none. Every test you have asks you to conform to a standard, an average, from which any deviation may be seen as cause for concern or for further observation.

This is an example of a mother who went on to have a perfectly normal home birth. She endured a stressful and roller-coaster pregnancy, which created unnecessary anxiety.

This mother was told that she was borderline for a home birth because she had a BMI (body mass index) of 30. She was fit and well and felt on balance that she was safer at home as it was where she felt comfortable and relaxed. She disliked hospitals and didn't want to birth her baby there; in fact she felt ill whenever she was near a hospital. Halfway through her pregnancy she was routinely tested for gestational diabetes. These tests have been introduced fairly recently; prior to this, women's urine was checked on a regular basis for sugar, which was seen as a possible indicator. She was borderline for gestational diabetes and told she would be unable to give birth at home. If she had been in the neighbouring hospital she would have been free to give birth at home within their policy. She continued to take readings at home, and never again showed an elevated reading after the test. At this point she was told that she might have to be induced early or have a Caesarean birth because of a potentially big baby and problems associated with gestational diabetes. The day she was scanned for the last time and checked at the hospital she was signed out of the diabetes clinic, but on the same day moved to another consultant who said that they suspected her baby was too small. The client was in a mixed-race relationship and knew that her husband's particular race was known to have small babies, yet this was not considered. It was suggested that she should be induced because her baby was too small. She paid for a private consultation to check the placental function and found that it was normal and the blood flow to baby was fine. She chose at that point, two weeks before her birth, to hire an independent midwife. She went on to have an undisturbed birth at home, with no pain relief or need for intervention. Her little girl was just under 6 lb and was perfect in every way.

CREATING YOUR BLANK BIRTH CANVAS

Once you understand the theory, you may think, 'I've got it! I know what to do.' However, this is where hypnosis preparation really differs from other forms of mind preparation. Whatever you think you know can differ from what your unconscious thinks it knows.

An automatic and instinctive fear response, triggered from what your unconscious thinks it knows, can override your conscious thoughts and trigger automatic responses in your body. This is particularly true of situations that you are unconsciously apprehensive or anxious about. Hypnosis is about resetting your automatic responses so your unconscious aligns with your healthy positive expectations and beliefs at a conscious level.

This is a really important element of understanding how hypnobirthing will work for you. The simplest way to help you understand how the dynamic works between the two different parts of your brain is to describe how a phobia develops over years but can be dissolved in hours. A phobia is an automatic fear-based response triggered by something that causes you anxiety. Understanding how a phobia is created will help you to understand why resetting your unconscious is so important when you want to have a gentle birth.

If you have a phobia or a fear of something, think about it now; put yourself in that position, knowing you are secure where you are, and allow yourself to get in touch with the feeling associated with that fear. You may be aware of some of the signs that your sympathetic nervous system has been activated – your heart may be beating a little faster, you may be breathing more rapidly, your palms may be sweaty.

As humans, our survival response has become a little muddled with mixed messages we receive around us, from the moment we are born right up until the present moment. Phobias are a result of this and are an automatic survival response in a situation where there is no need for us to go into survival mode.

Phobias can be triggered by things people have seen or heard: in films, on television, online and in the news. In one of my classes two men had phobias of deep water. I suggested that a phobia like that might have started when watching a film like *Jaws* at a young age. It could have been many things but both men said it had indeed started after they had watched *Jaws* and got progressively worse. This shows how powerful the messages around us in society can be.

Phobias and anxieties are interesting because people have an instinctive response to something they know will not harm them. People with phobias are very aware of this and often feel silly for reacting as they do, but are unable to stop themselves. Phobias can even stop people doing things they want to do, like flying or going down an escalator.

When Anna was six months old her mother − the person who loved, cared for and protected her − saw a spider, screamed and jumped on a chair. Anna saw the eight-legged creature in the corner of the room, recognised that her mother was afraid of the spider, so is likely to have formed a pattern in her brain that tells her house spiders can hurt her and are dangerous. From that moment on her fear may have been compounded each time she saw a spider until she was the one jumping on the chair screaming. Anna knew that the spider would not hurt her, that it was harmless, but her body took over.

The good news is that you can shift a phobia or an anxiety in a rapid amount of time − it's like pressing the reset button.

Resetting your Birth Brain

Imagine your brain as a map, with neurons connecting different parts of your brain, like roads going to destinations on the map. Your map is unique, and the routes and destinations are changing all the time based on experiences around you. When you were born your brain was already laying down routes, destinations and pathways on your own unique map, which impact on how you respond to your environment in your individual way. This brain mapping takes place at a rapid pace between birth and the age of three, then starts to slow down but remains very fast until the age of about 13. It's during this period that most of our automatic responses to the world around us are formed, and we are at our most impressionable.

Sometimes referred to as 'brain plasticity', this ability to change pathways in your brain is active into old age. So the good news is that you are still able to change your routes, destinations and pathways relating to any situations or destination, including your reactions to birth. Resetting your birth brain is simply making new routes in your brain and changing your reference system, so the route you take to birth is a different and better one. Although it may have taken years to establish a fear, anxiety or phobia, it can take as little as an hour to reset that thought.

LETTING GO OF YOUR FEARS

Your current reference system may look a little like this, which is consistent with how our thoughts around birth may be formed in our culture and society:

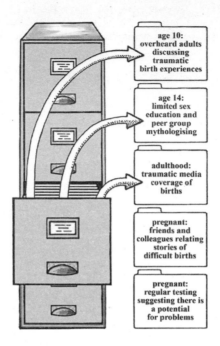

age 10:
overheard adults
discussing
traumatic
birth experiences

age 14:
limited sex
education and
peer group
mythologising

adulthood:
traumatic media
coverage of
births

pregnant:
friends and
colleagues relating
stories of
difficult births

pregnant:
regular testing
suggesting there is
a potential
for problems

*Trust that you can let go of anything from your past that
may cause your body to instinctively react in fear.*

Imagine clearing those files out, shredding the ones you wish to. Take a moment to dispose of those files in a way that feels right to you. Then think about where you might get positive messages about birth: friends who have had great experiences; an online support group consistent with mindful hypnobirthing; a family member; or a midwife you particularly like. Perhaps there are books that will help you to reshape your instinctive responses to birth so they are based on trust and the ability of your body to birth your baby. Take a moment to think about things that you could do to populate your reference system and write them in.

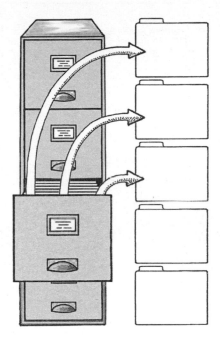

Fill your unconscious with positive things about birth.
Then actively choose to do what's on this list.

Another method of doing this is through a light mindfulness meditation on those thoughts. Imagine having the freedom to let go of any negative thoughts or feelings around birth. In this moment you are aware that everything you have been told around birth from other people is based on their experiences, not yours. Anything that has happened in the past that you have experienced is specific to a unique set of circumstances and can remain in the past.

Imagine that right now you have the power to change anything that happens in the future by letting go of anything that may cause you to react with fear. You can enjoy your pregnancy and birth in the present moment with calm excitement, trusting your body and your ability to birth your baby in your uniquely normal way.

Find somewhere where you can sit quietly for 15 minutes, breathing in and breathing out, establishing a rhythm and getting comfortable. Imagine with your outbreath that you are blowing out all your fears and worries. They may be things you are consciously aware of, or you can give your unconscious permission to let go of anything that is troubling you or making you anxious. Sometimes they may be symbols that come up; if so, that's fine, just let them go. Your imagination will do what's right for you.

Then imagine blowing them into a cloud and allowing that cloud to then drift away on a gentle breeze, leaving a clear blue sky. Continue to do this until you are just breathing in and breathing out, feeling lighter and clear of thoughts, just being with your breath.

The space you are creating is allowing room for new positive thoughts to come in and take root. You can do this once, or as often as you feel the need to. It can be a useful exercise if something or someone has unsettled you. It can also be useful during labour to let go of any fears that may arise at certain points of labour.

SUMMARY

- Let go of your fears around birth and the expectation of pain.
- Clear negative references to birth and open your mind to positive messages.
- Decide how you want to experience birth.
- It's time to create positive and healthy beliefs around birth to take you forward on your birth journey.

6

CREATING POSITIVE BIRTH BELIEFS

Even if it has not been your habit throughout your life so far,
I recommend that you learn to think positively about your body.

Ina May Gaskin, midwife

You've let go of your fear and created your blank canvas on which you are able to rewrite your birth map. From this moment onwards you will need to be sure that the messages you receive, both from yourself and from others, carry the message of a positive birth and that they are consistent with the type of birth you want.

This done in three ways:

1. Learning how the internal messages you give yourself form a belief that can help or hinder your birth – and how to change them.
2. Understanding the way you receive information from your environment.
3. Filling up your birth reference system with healthy, positive images of birth.

WILL YOUR INTERNAL BELIEFS
HINDER OR HELP YOU?

Take a moment to reflect on your tree in Chapter 3 and the type of birth you wish to have. Do your beliefs support that goal and are they consistent with the type of birth you want? Look into your heart: do you believe that you can have an empowering, positive birth experience? Do you believe that your body can do it? Do you believe you have choice? Do you believe that your baby is the perfect size for your body? Do you believe that birth is a normal, natural event, not a medical event?

How we think things are going to happen can be a self-fulfilling prophecy. Belief shapes action and action shapes experience. Richard Wiseman, a well-known psychologist, found that people who believed they were lucky *were* luckier because they saw opportunities for luck.

A Buddhist nun described it to me in this way:

> *When you have a garden in which weeds grow, our tendency is to water that garden with circular thoughts focused on that pain and suffering so the weeds continue to grow, taking nutrients from the soil and stopping flowers from growing and blooming. But if we stop nourishing those weeds with our thoughts, if we change our thinking, they will die off and flowers will have the space to grow freely, creating the space for something new.*

The beliefs that you have can be either destructive or constructive in nature. They come from a place of love and acceptance or of fear. Your thinking about birth can shape your experience of being pregnant and giving birth. If your beliefs support a mindful hypnobirth, it is likely that your experience will be a more positive one; if they don't, you are creating challenges to your hypnobirthing goal and setting doubt in your mind that you can do it. This understanding of how our internal belief systems work has been tested in various experiments and is known scientifically as 'selective attention' or the 'cocktail party effect'.

If you go to a party that's busy and a bit noisy, you may be standing chatting to someone and then suddenly you hear a friend's name or a place of work mentioned by someone around you. Amidst all the noise your brain picks up that information. What a coincidence, you think! In fact, your brain is processing and deleting information all the time like a filter. Any information that was irrelevant to you was already filtered out before it reached your conscious awareness.

Believe that Birth Can Be Great

Building up a positive belief is down to changing the way you think about birth. Once you have done that you'll change the messages you receive, both unconsciously and consciously, about birth. When you have a positive belief, your brain will filter through information that will reinforce that belief. Think of it as 'resetting your filter'. Suddenly you'll start seeing stories of great births, blogs, memes, television shows, empowering experiences and opportunities to share hints and tips relating to undisturbed birth and less and less about trauma.

Changing a belief means you have to begin to take active steps to make a change until it becomes a habitual part of your birth preparation. The external messages you receive and internal messages you give yourself have to support your goal of a mindful hypnobirth.

CHANGING EXTERNAL MESSAGES

Changing the messages you receive from your external environment is not as easy as changing internal beliefs, but it's easier than you might think to take practical steps to alter the information you receive. Of course we can't control everything in our environment, but even the things we can't control we can reframe. Reframing is simply taking a negative thought and turning it into a positive one.

If you experience something that upsets you or makes you question your ability to birth, use these questions to change negative messages into more positive ones:

1. According to whose perspective and what evidence?
2. What might be useful in this experience to me? What can I learn?
3. What would I say to a close friend in this situation?
4. What would I do now if I were having the mindful hypnobirth that I know I have the potential to have?

The sense of perspective is really important when observing others' experiences. Midwives often say they'll see what they think is a great birth and the mother will think it was awful. On the other hand, another woman may have had what a midwife would consider a difficult birth, but in reality the woman will have had a very positive experience.

Stand back and remember that information you are given is very often about belief and perspective. Give yourself the space to change your beliefs and your interpretation of birth as it's presented to you.

Five Quick and Easy Steps to Positive Messages

1. Change the Books you Choose to Read

There are so many books available for pregnancy. Among the more general pregnancy books, there are plenty which teach women about their bodies and birth in an empowering way. Take the time to research books and find at least one that gives you the messages you need to hear, which are aligned with your goals. Read a book that teaches you about your amazing body, gives you confidence to trust your body and to have patience in birth. See the Resources section on page 232 for recommended reading – books which women have told me were invaluable in changing their perspective on birth.

2. Stop Watching Adrenaline-fuelled Births on Television

Many programmes show women giving birth. Bear in mind that these will be edited so think about perspective and information. Often we don't have the full facts about what we are watching. Perhaps an edited show even reflects the editor's beliefs. Often producers of popular documentaries and writers of television shows want dramatic attention-grabbing storylines, rather than showing gentle, quiet births. Watching births on television can often skew your perception of birth. For example, fathers sometimes worry that their baby might be born en route to hospital, when this actually happens very rarely and makes headlines if it does. If you want to watch a birth that is consistent with a mindful hypnobirth, ask a friend to filter some out on YouTube for you to watch or find a Facebook page or blog that regularly posts positive stories.

3. Find Supportive Online Forums

Some online forums are hotbeds of what might go wrong. Find a forum that supports hypnobirthing. There are plenty out there. These forums will share information about positive births and it's always helpful to be around women who are supporting your birth choices.

4. Choose the Birth Stories you Wish to Hear

Instead of listening to a colleague's traumatic birth story when you are eight months pregnant you can choose to say, 'I really don't need to hear this right now.' You'll often find that women who have had normal, positive experiences, don't actually talk a lot about them. I've often heard women say, 'I didn't want to appear smug when everyone around me seemed to have such awful stories to tell.' If you have a friend who has had a very straightforward birth – ask her about it!

5. Attend a Class Focused on Positive Birth

There are many classes now that prepare women in a proactive way for an undisturbed birth, with yoga, active birth, doula-led classes, relaxation and hypnosis. Some women choose not to attend classes if they know that the focus is going to be on pain and intervention. It's not uncommon for some more conventional classes to still show you the forceps or an epidural needle, which of course would introduce you to the suggestion and belief of intervention and medical assistance.

You will also meet other pregnant women who are seeking out a similar experience to you, and this is incredibly helpful in supporting you on your journey. If you can't afford a class or don't have the time, look for a positive birth group near you. These have sprung up all over the world and hold meetings regularly that support women in having a positive birth. They are often well resourced, with books, films and information that can help reinforce a positive belief that you are designed to birth your baby, and that you can do it and enjoy the experience.

CHANGING INTERNAL MESSAGES

The first rule of internal messaging is 'be kind to yourself' and be your own best birth friend. Changing a belief is about stopping the cycle of negative thinking that would allow fears to grow again. Support yourself with gentle reminders that you can do this; your body is designed to birth your baby and women all over the world give birth every day and have a positive experience. You can be one of those women.

Over the next seven days, turn your awareness to the messages you give yourself about birth. Imagine that you are your best friend and supporting yourself in your mindful hypnobirth journey. Each time you have a negative thought, or a doubt slips into your mind, stop yourself, observe that thought and turn it into a positive thought.

BIRTH AFFIRMATIONS

Another way of changing your beliefs is to change the messages you give yourself about birth using affirmations. I have written a selection below, but change them around so that they feel like something you would say and then write them out yourself; this creates ownership of them. Place them somewhere in your home or at work where you can see them regularly. Say them twice a day at least.

If you have a specific loop of thought which goes around in your head, write an affirmation that counteracts that fear. For example, if you are worried about tearing at the birth write, 'As I relax and let go, following my breath, my body softly expands allowing the perfect-sized space for my baby to slip through.' Make sure that each affirmation is a positive statement.

Affirmations for You

1. I know that my body is designed perfectly to bring my baby into the world.
2. I trust and tune in to my birth instincts.

3. As my body grows I enjoy each change knowing that my body is creating the perfect temporary home for my baby.

4. The closer I get to my baby's birth date the more relaxed I am.

5. The more relaxed I am the easier it is to feel confident and in control.

6. When I go into labour I will relax quickly and easily into my rhythm.

7. I trust that I will know the perfect time to go into hospital/call the midwife.

8. With each contraction wave I will be more and more relaxed.

9. I'm excited but calm as I look forward to my baby's birth.

10. I know that my body is designed to soften and expand during labour.

11. The more I relax the more my body will soften and expand.

12. The more I soften and expand the more quickly my baby will come into the world.

13. Each contraction wave will bring my baby closer to being born.

14. Labour can be intense but I know that I can do it.

15. I am looking forward to welcoming my baby into the world.

16. I trust that I will be a wonderful mother.

Write your own …

Affirmations can also be helpful for the birth partner. Ask them to join you in writing out your affirmations together and talking about how you want to experience your birth.

Affirmations for your Birth Partner

These can also be helpful in developing the birth partner's confidence, not only as a birth partner but also in trusting that mum will know what to do.

1. I am a loving, gentle and kind birth partner.
2. As my partner grows and our baby grows I am in awe of how nature works.
3. I trust that my partner will instinctively know what to do when birth begins.
4. I will allow her the space to follow her instincts.
5. I will be patient, calm and loving.
6. I will be aware of my own fears and will set them aside for the birth.
7. With each contraction wave I will be strong, still and calm with my partner.
8. I will feel confident in communicating our preferences to the midwife.
9. I am excited about meeting my baby and becoming a father.

Write your own ...

SIT BACK, RELAX AND LET HYPNOTIC SUGGESTION DO IT FOR YOU

Listen to your hypnosis tracks every day as directed in the practice guidelines on page 37. There is an initial 30-minute track that will take you into a very deep state of hypnotic relaxation, and there are two other tracks, one of your pregnancy affirmations and one of your birth affirmations. The hypnosis suggestions will change your thinking at a deep level as you relax and enjoy letting go.

Suggestions are sometimes very obvious and sometimes more subliminal, but they are designed in a very specific way that allows your unconscious mind to adopt and own those beliefs. At the end of the day, it's you who has to allow those beliefs to take root; I'm just helping you sow the seeds. I know that you will be able to make these changes quickly and easily because you are reading this book and your intention is to change your thinking so you change your experience of birth. This is done so subtly that you might not even be consciously aware of the changes. You might just feel lighter, happier and calmly excited about the birth of your baby.

> **TIP:** It can be helpful to get yourself some good headphones and get used to wearing them. They are great at cutting out external disturbances and noise. The hypnosis tracks also use what's known as a dual induction. This works on stereo headphones and takes you very quickly and deeply into hypnosis.

SUMMARY

- Think about how your beliefs shape your experience. Remember, beliefs are learned from past experiences and based on their own unique circumstances.
- Your birth will be different from every other birth before you.
- Choose beliefs that support your mindful hypnobirth journey, then take time to reinforce and find information that supports that belief.
- Make sure that you read your affirmations and listen to your hypnosis tracks daily.

7

THE POWER OF VISUALISATION FOR BIRTH

The mind is everything. What you think you become.

Buddha

Visualisations and symbols are very powerful during pregnancy and birth; they are a connection with our unconscious – the part of our mind that extends beyond logic and reason. Visual symbols are connected with our creative right brain, which is also the home of our old brain, and tap deep into our being.

Traditionally, visualisations are associated with parts of our being that cannot be expressed through words. Language is a left brain function; sometimes it's hard to find words to express how we are feeling. However, we can try to think of that feeling as a colour or shape, or point to where it is in our body, perhaps turning it into a visual representation. This may make it much easier to get in touch with that feeling and to change it to something different and better.

The most important thing about a visualisation is the way in which your body responds to it. Previously, 'the power of visualisation' was thought to be a new age concept, but evidence now shows that when we imagine something it stimulates the part of the brain that is activated as if we were really performing that action. If I were to ask you to describe the colour yellow right now, the part of your brain that would be activated would be the part that would actually see the colour yellow. Studies show that athletes who visualise jumping higher in the high jump actually do. Visualisations associated with softness, expansion, confidence and calm relaxation can be very useful during labour and have true power to change how we respond to an experience physically.

The body responds to and physically mirrors visual images very effectively. Take the image of a flower opening, a birth image that has been around for years in cultures all over the world. This is symbolic of the body opening and softening and the cervix dilating. I use it sometimes as a visualisation during labour and it works beautifully to help a birth progress, where perhaps it had slowed down. With a client who is home birthing, I sometimes suggest having a bunch of flowers in the room that make her think of her body unfolding. Peonies are a popular choice.

Think of a flower you like and search YouTube for a time-lapse video of that flower. Watch it unfolding, paying attention to your body and directing your awareness to those very subtle shifts associated with that experience. The more you do it the more you will tune in to those shifts and changes. Be patient and give yourself time to become aware of how your body softens and relaxes in your pelvic area as the flower gently opens.

Another image that can be very popular during labour is of a woman expanding, or holding open, a very wide vagina. In their writing, Ina May Gaskin and Sheila Kitzinger often speak of

Sheela Na Gig, a form of gargoyle that can be found in Ireland and across Europe, which some anthropologists suggest helped fertility or birthing. A visual image that suggests this can do amazing things to your body. Here is one below that is similar to the idea of Sheela Na Gig.

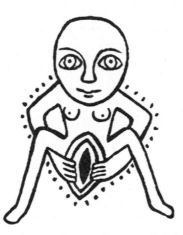

Your body is expansive. Let go of any conditioned responses that make you tense up, and embrace your body's ability to soften and expand.

YOU CAN CHANGE WHAT YOU FEEL

You can also use visualisations to alter perceptions of sensations in your body. In hypnosis for pain management, a sensation dial is commonly used to turn down sensations or feelings. Think back to page 58 when I talked about interpretations of sensation. This visualisation allows you to choose which sensation you wish to feel and at what intensity.

Choose where you want to place the dial. Then set the second dial to the intensity of sensation you wish to feel, with 10 being the strongest and 0 being nothing at all.

Birthing Barometer
turning down any pain

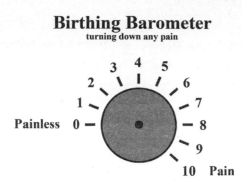

Draw your own arm on the dial, and point it to the intensity of sensation you wish to experience during birth. Then close your eyes and picture it in your head, moving it to where you wish it to be. You can imagine this during birth to turn down sensations.

Sensation Dial

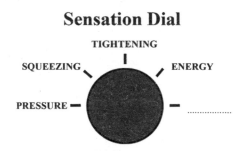

Draw your own arm on the dial, pointing to how you would want to experience the sensation of birth, or even write your own sensation.

Copy them out or cut them out, and put them up somewhere in your home where you will see them regularly. The more often you see the image, the easier it becomes to recall that image during birth. If you were to recall the dials during birth, you could imagine moving the dial up and down according to what you are experiencing in that moment. For example, you would be able to turn a sensation down or even numb that sensation. You can practise this if you hurt yourself at all, get cramps or even stub your toe!

TIP: Practise changing sensations for birth by getting an ice cube and putting it on a sensitive part of your arm, like your elbow or wrist. Set a timer to one minute, which is about as long as a contraction. Focus on your breathing and then imagine the dials; imagine turning that sensation down, changing the feeling of that sensation. You can also do this with your partner by asking them to hold the ice cube while you use this visualisation. Try this while listening to your hypnosis tracks to get used to how well hypnosis works. The more you practise, the easier it gets, and the easier it gets, the easier it is to apply during labour.

CREATING YOUR OWN VISUALISATION

You can create your own visualisation to use during labour that automatically relaxes your muscles, making you feel secure, familiar and happy. Your body will respond in a positive way because it will respond as if it were really there. For example, if I were to ask you to close your eyes right now, imagine your last holiday and describe it to me, I'm sure that your muscles would relax, your shoulders drop and you would get a sense of wellbeing associated with recalling your holiday.

Spend some time with your partner or a friend who can write down the story of your special place. Sit somewhere quiet where you are relaxed, focusing on your breathing. Close your eyes. Allow your mind to bring you to a place, somewhere you may have been to in the past or somewhere that you go to, and where you feel relaxed and calm. If you are doing this with your partner they shouldn't ask what you feel, see or hear, but should just say, 'Tell me about your place,' 'Tell me more,' and write down exactly what you say. Perhaps just get yourself relaxed and write it out yourself; do what feels right for you. Then relax yourself to the music or with your breathing and have your partner read that story back to you. You'll relax very quickly, your brain filling in the experience internally. Experiment with your partner recording their voice over the music so that you can listen to your calm story and get used to how it feels for you. You can use the background music download mentioned in this book. Alternatively, you can choose a sound you particularly like, such as waves if your visualisation is on a beach.

TIP: I use this if the woman I am with needs a rest. It can be particularly useful in long early labours or while you are waiting for an induction to begin working. Lie on your left side, put the background track on and have your partner read your story to you. Your mind will fill in any blanks as you drift off to your place; you may even fall asleep. An hour of this can be a great recuperation; your contractions may even get stronger without you realising.

Create a Birth Board

It is really helpful to collect images or phrases that you will find supportive during labour. Even better, create a 'birth board' where you can display your collection. You could do this by using a wall at home. If you want to bring your collection to the hospital, use a piece of card. As you progress in your mindful hypnobirthing practice, you will find that you gravitate more towards some phrases or images. Create little Post-its or posters of them and have them around you.

The image of a baby surfing worked very well for one of my clients. Whenever she looked at it, she was reminded of her baby being brought to her by the waves. Think about the Sheela Na Gig image (see page 81), or an image of a large flower opening. Another client of mine had what she called her 'oxytocin photos' – pictures of her with her daughter and her husband which made her feel happy.

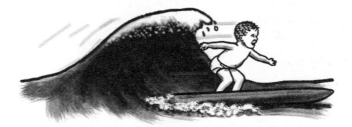

Imagine your baby surfing each contraction.

I FIND IT HARD TO VISUALISE – WILL IT STILL WORK FOR ME?

Even if you struggle to picture something, you can *imagine* something. Personally, I can't picture a dial in my head very well; however, I sense it and I can feel myself turning my dial down. Often a hypnotherapist will use the word 'imagine' instead. This allows you to conjure up an impression of a place or an image in a way that makes sense to you.

Everybody can imagine, and most people can visualise if they practise. Close your eyes and recall a place you love, outside in the country or at a beach. Be aware of how it is when you recall that place. Spend five minutes resting and imagining you are there. You may not have been able to visualise it, but however you did it, you would be able to access that place, the feelings and emotions associated with it.

One woman I was working with was frightened of being in hypnosis. She had come to me as a referral from a trusted friend, and said she wasn't visual at all. I just asked her to sit there with her eyes open and tell me about her last holiday, until I could see her start to relax. Then I asked her to close her eyes, which would bring it back in even more detail. After she'd finished she realised that in fact she could imagine a place and its detail in her own way. This gave her the confidence to continue exploring other ways of visualising.

SUMMARY

- Get creative – start thinking about how visualisations can help you during birth.
- Collect images that you can take to the birth with you as visual reminders to help you relax and let go in your body and mind.
- Spend time creating your own visualisation for birth, asking your partner to help.

8

YOUR BIRTH BELONGS TO YOU

You are constructing your own reality with the choices you make ... or don't make. If you really want a healthy pregnancy and joyful birth, and you truly understand that you are the one in control, then you must examine what you have or haven't done so far to create the outcome you want.

Kim Wildner

In this chapter, we'll explore a little more about choice and control. Many women I speak to are not aware of their choices and feel out of control during pregnancy and as they approach birth. You may feel overwhelmed with information or that you are not getting enough of the information you want in order to make your choices around birth.

Your relationship with your midwife is important. Being familiar with different models of care will help you to organise your thinking around your birth preferences and know what to expect. This can help you make more considered decisions on the day of your baby's birth.

WHO SUPPORTS YOU IN YOUR BIRTH?

The first and most positive thing about UK maternity care is that the majority of women are cared for by a midwife (midwifery-led care). This differs in other countries like the US where each woman is assigned an obstetrician who will make decisions about her care. Studies show that the advantage of midwifery-led care is that you are at lower risk of intervention and much more likely to have an undisturbed birth.

Over the past 30 years the emphasis has shifted from a focus on continuity of care to a model where women are often unfamiliar with the person who will help them at the birth of their baby. You may have the same midwife when you go to your antenatal appointments, or you may have a different midwife each time. How you are cared for depends largely on where you live. You may be lucky enough to have what's known as continuity of care, and a case-loading midwife. This means that the same midwife will support you through your pregnancy and birth, and also postnatally.

If you choose to give birth in hospital, even if you have been lucky enough to have the same midwife through all your antenatal appointments, you are likely to have a completely different midwife caring for you through your birth. If you have a home birth you may have a midwife you've met in your antenatal clinic, but this is dependent on shifts, as community midwives work a rota of being on call.

Preparing Your Birth Choices

Women and men I've worked with are understandably cautious about giving someone they've never met the responsibility of caring for them, when the mother may be at her most vulnerable, physically and emotionally. Not only that but you also have to entrust your birth preferences to them, something you may have carefully reflected on over the last few months, choosing how you wish to welcome your baby into the world. A trusting relationship with the midwife is essential in feeling supported, cared for and safe, and recognising that your birth choices will be respected.

Working closely with your community midwife to explore your options and choices can be very helpful. If you are planning a mindful hypnobirth, you may have already begun to feel more positive about how you are in control of mental processes, which can allow labour to progress well. You may also be considering things that you previously had not. You may feel more strongly about certain elements of your birth and more aware of how you wish to explore other options.

Your community midwife will help you to explore information and research that support your choices, and be able to signpost you to other organisations that can help you. If you feel that your community midwife isn't being as helpful as you'd like (remember many of them are under a lot of stress and pressure to move appointments along), ask for a double appointment next time to discuss things in more detail. If you feel your wishes aren't being supported you can request an appointment with the supervisor of midwives. This is especially useful if you have a choice that may challenge conventional policies and guidelines in your hospital area. Supervisors of midwives are very experienced and are there to help support you in the birth you want; they are also able to help write your preferences. They can ensure that any requests you have are written down and agreed before the birth.

You may also like to consider hiring a doula to help you navigate your choices, and support you through your pregnancy and birth.

What's a Doula?

A doula is a trained birth attendant who can offer you continuity of care. She will visit you before the birth, be with you during the birth from when you need her, and also sometimes postnatally.

A doula becomes a familiar companion, someone who can support you, your partner and your choices. She can allow you to completely let go during the birth, feeling safe in the knowledge that you have the support of a trusted independent birth companion. Research shows that attendance of a doula can reduce intervention by up to 50 per cent and improve birth outcomes. You can hire a doula either through Doula UK, which is a regulating body, or through the National Childbirth Trust (NCT) who train 'Birth Companions'.

A doula will chat to you about how you wish her to support you and your partner. It may be that she is the main emotional support while the father does the practical work:

Our doula was amazing and was there every step of the way giving me support. Words cannot express how I feel about the support I received. Our doula kept me calm and relaxed and was my main support throughout labour. She also supported my husband and kept him focused on filling the pool and calling the midwife. She showed love and support and was born to be a doula. I will never forget how special she is and the support she gave.

You may prefer your doula to do the practical things in the birthing environment so your partner can focus on being the emotional support:

It was just how we had planned and exactly what I had spent weeks hoping for. I had a quick and beautiful birth, so much of which was down to our doula's help. Even my husband says she transformed the delivery room into a calming place. I think her just being there changed the atmosphere. I will never forget my birth experience for all the right reasons.

If you are worried about the expense, there is a UK Doula Access fund for some women. Also, if a doula has just trained she charges only expenses until she attends four births.

WHAT DOES BEING IN CONTROL MEAN TO YOU?

Control is an interesting concept when it comes to birth. What does it actually mean to you? Is it control of how you physically respond to birth? In our culture we are taught to be self-restrained, to control ourselves physically and to keep a stiff upper lip, often not openly showing emotion or feeling. You may hold concerns about whether you are in control of the process and of your birth choices.

Think carefully about why it is important that you are in control of your birth. What control means to you is fundamental to understanding how to prepare yourself and those supporting you. Although many women say, 'I'm afraid of losing control,' this means something different to every woman and will mean something specific to you. Beneath this response lies a tapestry of fears and apprehensions connected to a woman's personal life experience and personality. Let's unravel it. There are three different forms of control during birth, which will be discussed in detail below:

1. Control of your choices.
2. Control of your environment.
3. Control of your physical reaction to birth.

Being in Control of your Choices and Environment

You may have already decided what type of birth you want. You may have thought carefully about the environment, how you want your baby to be received, whether you want to avoid unnecessary intervention. There are many choices you can make in your preparation and include in your birth preferences.

Those supporting an 'undisturbed birth' will say, 'If mum's fine and baby's fine then do nothing.' In many cases, when labour slows down or a mother isn't progressing as quickly as the midwife or doctor may wish, intervention is offered in line with hospital policy so it's worth familiarising yourself with local policies. In fact, there are usually many other options and alternatives to try first which may prevent intervention.

Policies and Guidelines – What's the Difference?

Policies and guidelines are different. How your midwife uses these may alter the course of your birth. A policy is a written document that outlines the exact requirements or rules that must be met in specific situations that may arise. It is a route of practice a midwife is obliged to take, unless a mother requests otherwise.

A guideline is a recommendation for best practice. Guidelines are not must-follow requirements. An experienced midwife I once knew said to me that 'guidelines are like tramlines' – you could step outside them, but often it was a midwife's own experience and trust in birth that gave her the confidence to do that, and tailor care to individual mothers. It may come down to an individual midwife's own way of practising which dictates how she navigates the guidelines.

You can do your own research around a policy and decline to comply with it. A midwife has to follow policy; you don't. One of the most basic principles of health care is that every patient (including pregnant women) has the right under common law to give or withhold consent to medical examination or treatment. However, it is worth knowing that although you can turn a policy-driven intervention down, there are some options that may be closed to you. For example, in a hospital certain facilities, such as the pool, may be off limits if you choose to go against policy.

A woman who was pregnant with her first baby was diagnosed with Group B Strep (GBS). She was told that she would have to have antibiotics and would not be able to use the birth pool. This was at a major teaching hospital in the UK. Using the pool was a big part of her birth preferences so her only choice was to have a home birth where she could hire her own pool. She wanted to be in hospital so she really did her research, and she found a robust and recent study that showed how a water birth significantly reduced the risk of transmission of infection to the baby. She wrote a letter referencing the research to the hospital. Although the hospital was unable to change the policy in time to allow her to use the pool in the hospital, she was able to negotiate a home birth with a pool. She received the antibiotics at the hospital and went home to birth. The hospital then went through the process of changing its official policy so that in future mothers could use the pool at the hospital.

Being offered an intervention means you have been offered a choice, not a decision. These are the times when it may seem difficult to know the right thing to do. It's often at these moments that women and their partners relinquish control and just say yes to the intervention offered without understanding the full implications.

UNDERSTANDING CHOICES ABOUT CARE

It's important to understand the psychology of how risk is communicated in a hospital setting. The concept of risk is complicated, and communicating the risk of an intervention in a birth situation does not always seem simple. There are many different factors which need to be taken into account. Studies on the psychological perception of risks show just how difficult this can be.

If you are using your emotional brain you are more likely to extract the general gist of any information to make your decisions, rather than really understanding the implications of the choice you are making. Decision-making is based on feeling, not fact, and our ability to be objective is sometimes challenged at birth, especially if we are frightened and anxious. Always take the time to ask about absolute risk, rather than relative risk, as this often gives you a much clearer understanding. For example, if your waters break before labour starts, you may be told that the risk of your baby getting an infection doubles after 24 hours; that's the relative risk. The research actually shows that the risk rises from around 0.5 per cent to around 1 per cent; that tells you the absolute risk and gives a much less frightening picture. So while the risk has increased, it's still very low. You may also be told the relative risks in association with induction so it's well worth asking for the absolute risk in order to make a balanced decision. If you don't understand something that your doctor is trying to tell you, ask them to draw a diagram; some obstetricians do this automatically, others don't. Studies show that people are able to process the information better this way and feel more informed.

If you are faced with a choice during the birth, take your time. Things sometimes happen much slower than you think; ask the doctor and the midwife to give you time to talk to your partner and to make a decision. As a doula I always say, 'Thanks for talking us through all the options. We'd like a few minutes to just reflect on them.'

Are you Ms Average or Ms Unique?

The journey of birth has been overlaid with clinical measurements based on averages when in reality the spectrum of possibilities at birth is enormous. From questions around length of pregnancy and how many centimetres women dilate over a certain period of time, through to the three stages of labour, all of these force birth into a model that doesn't fit perfectly for anyone.

Applying measurements to labour makes it easy to fall into the trap of thinking that you should be meeting certain targets through your labour and, if you don't, you have somehow failed and need help. This is where control is taken away, because although women know at a deep level that they can do this, and they don't need someone else to do it for them, there is always the implicit suggestion that something is wrong if they don't meet those 'targets'.

You may be thinking, 'I'm not a medical expert, I don't know all the answers.' This may be true, but it's also true that even experts – whatever field they work in – get stuck in routines and habits. I heard a doctor once say that when he worked on obstetrics and gynaecology and was faced with a situation where a mother wasn't progressing, he would first ask which consultant the mother was under, as he knew that the management would be different with each consultant. Every doctor and every midwife may deal with any given situation in a different way, based on their experience and their training.

Being prepared, and understanding what the most basic interventions are, can help but your midwife is an expert. She is the person who can help and support you to make the choices that will allow you to have the birth you want, to feel in control and, importantly, to have a positive experience whatever path your birth takes. A good midwife can step outside the guidelines when she knows what you want, still keeping you and your baby safe. She recognises that you aren't Ms Average, and that your birth can be totally unique but perfectly normal.

How Do I Make the Right Decision?

It can be reassuring to have prepared a series of questions to ask your midwife or caregiver, should you be offered an intervention. I always equip mothers and their birthing partner with a BRAINS handout (see opposite). If offered an intervention, first of all always ask, 'Am I well?' and 'Is my baby well?' If so, you can ask the other questions that follow. Your priority, of course, is to ensure that you and the baby are well.

Ideally, your partner should practise asking these questions so that they are able to support you fully and ask as many as possible on your behalf. You may be centred in your birthing zone, and if there is no medical indication for an intervention your birth partner will be able to have that conversation and buy time without you having to come out of your zone. You should also be confident that your partner understands what you want as a couple. Remember, in order to allow your body to do what it does naturally, you have to shut down the thinking part of your brain, and having a partner, trusted friend or doula that can ask questions for you is ideal.

> **TIP:** Don't ever feel pressured into making a decision on the spot. This is when people make decisions they regret. Ask the midwife or the doctor to leave the room while you have some time to discuss it. Even if you need intervention, knowing you have reached that decision through informed choices and have been part of that decision process means you can have a fulfilled and positive birth experience.

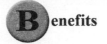 **B**enefits

What are the benefits of this intervention to the mother and baby?

What are the benefits to the baby?

 Risks

What are the risks of this intervention to the mother and baby?

How could my labour change if we have this intervention?

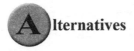 **A**lternatives

What alternatives could we try first? (We would like to keep intervention at a minimum)

We would like to keep this birth as undisturbed as possible. Do you have any suggestions?

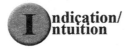 **I**ndication/ntuition

What's the indication for this intervention, are you concerned about the baby or the mother?

Is there a medical reason for this intervention?

If mum's fine and baby's fine then we'd rather wait.

Can we wait another hour, if all is well?

What's your intuition telling you? Use your breathing and self-hypnosis to tune into your body. Very often women during labour say that they 'just knew' what to do.

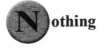 **N**othing

What would happen if we did nothing?

If mum is doing well and baby is showing no signs of distress we'd like to do nothing and wait a while.

We'd like time to think about it.

If all is well we'd like to do nothing and stay with our birth choices a little longer.

If labour has slowed down or stopped, can we go home for a bit?

 Smile

Ask everything gently, softly, with a smile! Building up good rapport with your midwife will help you both feel calmer and encourage a sense of cameraderie, familiarity and trust.

You can print this sheet out at www.mindful-hypnobirthing.co.uk.
Keep it with you in hospital and refer to it if you need a reminder.

WILL YOU ROAR LIKE A LIONESS
OR BE QUIET AS A CAT?

During birth, it's important to know that it's okay to make a noise and it's okay to be quiet or silent. Our fear of losing physical control is connected to our sense of self-awareness, a very human trait, which is an obstacle when it comes to birth. In Chapter 4 you learned about the role of the neo-cortex – the thinking part of your brain – and by now you should be aware of how important it is to create an environment that allows this part of the brain to quieten down.

You are in control of allowing yourself to let go, and can make the choices that are important to creating an environment in which you feel safe, private and unwatched. The trust you have in your birthing partner to maintain that sense of safety and privacy for you is very important. You also need to feel safe with the people present in the birth room, and that they are not judging you.

Sometimes we find ourselves in situations that are new or unfamiliar. It's at these times when we may be most conscious of being judged and watched. This heightened sense of feeling watched is pronounced during birth. The result can be an unconscious physical tension and 'holding back', creating a fear of letting yourself go. Michel Odent, a well-known French obstetrician, believes that a woman has to let go of the need to be in control in order to birth; she has to surrender to the experience of birth.

Sarah J. Buckley writes that:

When we birth consciously, putting our great rational mind on hold and allowing our instinctive nature to dominate, we can access a wisdom that all spiritual traditions teach; that the ego is our servant, not our mistress, and that our path to ecstasy and enlightenment involves surrendering our egoistic notions of control. This level of surrender will also serve us well through our many years of motherhood.

Both Buckley and Odent elaborate on the need to surrender to the experience with acceptance and to have faith in yourself and in birth.

Crucially, you have to know that you are in control of the choice to let go and to allow yourself the opportunity to have your best birth the way that you want to express it. It shouldn't matter what anyone else thinks; this is a time to have the confidence to know that you can let go, make noise, be quiet and move in any way you wish to, unhindered by anxiety or embarrassment.

It's a commonly held belief that hypnobirthing mums are quiet and calm, and they often are. Women who see themselves as calmer instinctively choose methods of birth preparation that create a more relaxed environment, and women using hypnosis techniques are calmer and more focused. I've heard midwives who attend hypnobirths say that sometimes they hardly notice when the mother moves into the final moments before her baby is born. These women may look as if nothing is happening to them, but if you talk to a woman afterwards, she will often tell you that on the contrary she was aware of her contractions but was deeply focused, present and in her zone.

Hypnobirthing mums can also make a lot of noise, and this is fine. Some women can find great rhythm through vocalising, or making sound with their out-breath. Often that surge of adrenaline as baby is soon to be born allows a mother to make a deep roar or projection of sound. This noise is deeply instinctive and primal. Some communities call it a birth cry. Midwives listen out for this and always run in when the mother starts making deep guttural growls!

TIP: If you are relaxed in your upper body, jaw and throat, sounds that you make should be low-toned, like humming, and may get softer or louder depending on the length or strength of the contractions. If your voice gets high-pitched or you begin to scream, open your mouth and take a deep breath. Just opening your mouth and taking a deep breath will relax your jaw and will bring the tone lower. It can be useful to have your partner do it too, as you will find that you mirror your partner.

SUMMARY

- You can make choices every step of the way, whatever path your birth takes.
- If you are higher risk and under consultant-led care you can make decisions about your care that will help you have a positive experience.
- Decide what and who you need to support your choices.
- Do your research on choices that are important to you, so that you can ask detailed questions.
- Remember, take your time having things explained to you fully so you can make an informed choice.

9

BIRTH PREFERENCES

I'm like a chameleon. Every woman is unique and for every woman that I care for I need to be a different midwife. I don't know how to be her perfect midwife unless she tells me.

Chantelle Thornley

I choose to use the term 'birth preferences' rather than 'birth plan', as you can't plan your birth. Preferences are about making sure that the midwife knows what you don't want, and things you absolutely do want.

You may have thought long and hard about your birth choices, but if you haven't written them down they may be forgotten. They become your road map to a new destination, and remind you of the route you have chosen; you can always check your map if you feel like you are going off course. Trying to negotiate logically on the day is very difficult because of the emotional intensity; it really helps to have a sheet with your birth preferences written out. This reminder is as important to you as it is to the midwife. It always surprises me when people are so keen to prepare well for the birth but don't have their preferences written down and slotted in the back of their notes.

If you are under a consultant, it's even more important to write your preferences down. Before the birth you can negotiate things such as pool use, reduced monitoring, or even the option to switch to midwifery-led care if all is well, but make sure that they are on your preferences. You may be surprised at how much you can prepare and what choices are available to you. I had one client who didn't want a forceps delivery under any circumstances. Her preferences stated that, in the event of a likely assisted delivery and if the baby seemed compromised, she wanted to go straight to a Caesarean birth. She had a discussion with her obstetrician beforehand so she didn't have to negotiate on the day, which can be very stressful and push you into making decisions you really don't want to make.

HOW TO WRITE MINDFUL HYPNOBIRTH PREFERENCES

Mindful hypnobirthing preferences are different to a straight-forward birth plan. The ones that I've helped women write over the years have been commented on many times by midwives, and I've more than once heard that it's one of the best birth plans they've read. This is because they are short, simple and tell them exactly what they can do to help the mum have the birth she wants.

The basic rules to stick to are:

- Keep it short (under a page).
- Bullet point it, so it's easy for the midwife to read if things happen quickly.
- Put what you don't want or are not sure about on the preferences (you can always change your mind later).
- Let the midwife know how she can help you.
- Keep three copies: two in your hospital bag so that you have a copy for you and an extra one in case you need to hand it to the midwives again. Always put one in the back of your notes, which will be given to the midwife.

- The birthing partner should take it out and go through it with her. I've done this often and found that the midwife hadn't read them or realised they were there.

The following suggestions are appropriate for an undisturbed birth but can also be applied to what may be considered a higher risk birth.

1. You have consent to listen to the baby's heart with a Doppler (an electrical device)/take my blood pressure/ temperature when you wish without having to ask me.

When you are hypnobirthing you need to make sure that the midwife knows you don't want to be disturbed all the time. For every intervention the midwife has to ask your permission; this includes listening to the baby's heart every 15–20 minutes. Imagine that you are in your birthing zone, focused and in tune with the rhythm of your body. Your neo-cortex is dampened down, and then the midwife comes in and asks if she can listen to the baby's heartbeat. Midwives are taught to build rapport with labouring mums – it's part of their training – and when they ask you to check the baby it's like a window of opportunity to verbally build rapport. I've seen naturally quiet midwives leap in and start asking mum lots of questions and try to make small talk. This can switch on your thinking brain, taking you out of your birthing zone and making you feel compelled to build conversation as our social conditioning tells us it's rude to ignore someone.

By writing the above statement on your birth preferences you can reduce interruptions by giving permission for the midwives to do their checks without having to ask you.

2. We would prefer a quiet midwife who is interested in undisturbed birth as we've prepared using hypnosis/ mindfulness/yoga.

Some midwives are more hands-on than others and like to be practical; they can be very helpful for mothers who are more afraid or need that interaction. Women who are prepared, feel comfortable and are using hypnobirthing often feel confident enough to just quietly be with their partner, knowing that they can call the midwife if they need her. Often, if you have this in your birth preferences you will attract a midwife who is interested in undisturbed birth. Birth preferences are often discussed at hand over, or when a couple comes in, so the right match of midwife can be assigned to you. Finding the right match of midwife for couples is important and is something that is commonly done in units where I've been at births. You can help them get it right by being clear about the type of midwife and birth you want.

3. Please don't offer me pain relief. I'll ask for it if I need it.

Think about it. You are in your birthing zone. You may be quietly breathing through each contraction or making noise, but you are focused in each moment. You may not even be aware that you are making any sound. Then someone asks if you want pain relief. This can trigger thoughts like, 'Is it going to get worse?' 'Do I look like I'm not coping?' Even if you are doing well and are focused, you are very likely to accept the pain relief without really thinking about it, even if you don't need it. This is because you are in a highly suggestible frame of mind when you are in your birthing zone.

Having this statement on your birth preferences tells your carers that you know pain relief is available and that you can ask for it.

4. If you are not sure about vaginal examinations then have something on your birth preferences. If you want to have

them and don't want to know the result then write that; or if you don't want them put that down. If you want one just as an initial assessment, then no more, have that on your preferences. If you are happy about having them as and when, just leave this off your plan.

If you don't want something, or you are not sure that you want it, put it in your preferences that you don't want it. Remember you can change your mind at any point and ask for an intervention such as a vaginal examination. This ensures that you are not pushed into doing anything you're unsure about and can make a decision based on whether it feels right for you at the time, not what is being suggested to you. You know that option is there and that you can ask.

5. We would like to approach this birth with patience. In the absence of any medical indications we would prefer to allow the birth to take its own time.

Mindful hypnobirthing is about allowing the birth to progress in its own time, having trust in a mother's ability to birth and, when both mum and baby are well, to let it be. Having this on your preferences tells the midwife that if all is well you would prefer to wait. In the absence of anything else, birth slowing down is not a medical indication for intervention, nor is slow dilation. Remember what you have learned in the book and use your head and your hypnosis to wait patiently for labour to start again. This is the point when women very often fall into intervention unwillingly.

6. Think about mentioning you want to follow your body's urge to push and not to have direction to push.

I've seen mothers breathe and breathe and breathe, and at the very last moment when they have the urge, push. It's very easy for people around a mother to get excited and carried away, making lots of noise and loudly encouraging the mother to push. Baby's nearly here after all; it *is* exciting. When I've seen mothers being told to push, I see them tense up. Your baby will come; follow your body and keep breathing. The more relaxed you are the more your muscles will soften and expand. You will feel your baby moving down and it is incredible. Women say that despite what they thought, this is in fact often the easiest part of their labour.

Many hospitals now have guidelines in place that allow a passive hour. This means just letting the mother follow her body, with no directions to push within that time. However, this isn't the case everywhere, so it's useful to have this in your notes if you want to be left to follow your body's lead.

7. Think about whether you would like a physiological third stage/cord to be left until it's stopped pulsating.

This is very important to have on your preferences if it's what you want; midwives will read this and take note. Managed third stages are routine in UK hospitals and mean that you are given medicine to help the uterus clamp down and release the placenta.

Usually, it's while you are holding your baby with your partner just after the birth. You will be focused on your baby, not on anything else, and the midwife may say somewhere in the background, 'Do you want something to help with the placenta?' She has to have your consent to give the syntocinon or syntometrine. You may absentmindedly agree because your focus is on your baby, not on what the midwife is saying. Before you know it you have a needle in your thigh and are having a managed third stage.

There is plenty of research and information about physiological third stages and managed third stages. Read up on it so you really understand what you are consenting to.

8. Keep the room quiet, dark and free of interruption after the birth. Think about immediate skin to skin contact, and no weighing for at least an hour.

This is such an important time, this first hour after birth. The birth isn't finished when the baby is born; it continues in those moments and hours after birth. Keeping the room quiet, dark and warm – much the same as for the birth – helps release the placenta and also makes the transition for the baby much gentler and less stressful. Baby's weight is not going to change much in that short time, and he or she will certainly find much more comfort snuggled up on your chest, next to the familiar beat of your heart, than on a cold hard set of scales in those minutes after birth. If your baby has to be taken off you for any reason, pass baby to your partner and ask him to just quietly talk to the baby. I've seen babies cry when they are taken off their mothers after being very calm and chilled but quickly settle in their father's arms after hearing his familiar voice.

TAILORING YOUR PREFERENCES TO YOUR LOCAL GUIDELINES

Other things to consider may be specific to the area you live in. For example, in some areas you may be put on a continuous monitor for 20 minutes when you arrive at the hospital, even if you are considered low risk and midwifery led, whereas other areas will monitor your baby at regular intervals. Some areas may be more likely to administer antibiotics to the baby after the birth. Some may allow a pool birth for some higher risk births, while others do not. It always amazes me how hospitals and midwives differ in their approaches. Understanding what the guidelines, policies and 'trends' in your local area are will give you a better idea of what to expect and how to prepare for it. Your midwife, or perhaps a local doula, will be able to help you with this.

TIP: Many groups across the UK are linked to an organisation called the Positive Birth Movement. These are often run by mothers, doulas or antenatal teachers who want to help mothers in their area have a positive experience. They will be very familiar with guidelines and policies local to you, and it's well worth getting in touch with your local group. You can find the website in the Resources section (see page 232).

SUMMARY

- Write your birth preferences at least four weeks before your due date.
- Attend a local group and try to meet other women who can tell you about local guidelines.
- Go through your preferences with your midwife or, if you want independent eyes on it, see if you can make a private appointment with a doula or an independent midwife.
- Make three copies, keep two in your birth bag and tuck one inside the maternity notes. If things happen quickly, this is the first place your carers will look.
- You or your partner should always go through your birth preferences with your midwife point by point when you meet her on the day.

10

BIRTH SPACE, RELAXING SPACE

It seems that there are two major differences between simple births and more painful ones. These differences concern the place where the mother gives birth and the position in which she does it.

Desmond Morris

The place where you give birth can influence the type of birth you have. Simply put, if you are in an environment where you feel secure, protected, cared for and familiar, your body responds well by releasing the hormone oxytocin, which promotes the willingness to give birth. The type of pregnancy you have, your own health and your expectations of birth may define your choice of birthing place.

It's generally expected that women will give birth in hospital. Although a midwife should ask you, 'Do you want to give birth at home or in hospital?' more often than not you'll hear, 'Which hospital do you want to have your baby in?' In the last few years, however, more women are making the decision to birth at home, and in some parts of the UK home birth rates have been rising.

Making an informed choice about where to give birth is the first step to taking ownership of your birth space. It really helps to understand the reasons why home births and hospital births differ and which is right for you. It's important that the choice you make is not based on fear but comes from a place of confidence and understanding. A decision made out of knowledge and confidence will allow you to adapt and relax into your birth space, knowing that you have chosen to be there.

In Chapter 5 you learned how your body reacts to unconscious fears or apprehension. You now know that oxytocin is a private hormone and that stress hormones react to unfamiliar, or potentially threatening, situations. When you are birthing it is very important to create an environment where you feel private and secure, with things that are familiar and comforting around you. This means that oxytocin flows and labour progresses well.

There are two things in our environment that we need to think about:

- What makes a great birth space?
- Who makes a birth space great?

WHAT MAKES A GREAT BIRTH SPACE?

There are very simple changes that you can make to any birth space which trigger unconscious muscle relaxation and a sense of familiarity. You relate to the world around you through your senses. Your brain filters information gathered from your senses, which then triggers rapid automatic responses via your personal reference system in your brain.

This is how your unconscious may turn your sensory input into an action or a feeling at birth. 'Hmmm, antiseptic smell, what does that remind me of? Ah, hospitals.' How you react or feel internally is dependent on what a hospital means to you. You may not like hospitals; you may work in one and feel at home; everyone reacts in a different way. The smell is known as an 'anchor' for that feeling or emotion.

Anchors

Anchors are things you can see, touch, hear, taste or smell that hold an emotional resonance. Think about the last time you went on holiday and perhaps a song, or a view you saw every day, or maybe something special you ate. Close your eyes and recall that memory; be aware of how your recall brings back a physical sense of being on that holiday again. You may even have noticeably relaxed, if it was a relaxing holiday!

Anchors are very easy to create; it's just about repeatedly attaching a feeling or an emotion to an object. Creating anchors specifically for your birth that trigger a sense of relaxation means that when you place the anchors in your birth space they trigger positive emotions and calm feelings deep within you, wherever you are. If you were in a busy shopping centre feeling anxious, and suddenly heard the music from your holiday, you might shift from a state of anxiety to a smile and a brief letting go. Learn what sensory challenges there may be in your birth environment but also how you can overcome them by using anchors to shift your senses into a state of calm relaxation. Imagine it as your own portable multi-relaxation system.

When thinking about creating the perfect birth space you need to consider:

- What you can see.
- What you can feel.
- What you can hear.
- What you can smell.

What You Can See

What you can see around you can trigger different feelings. For example, the resuscitation unit in the corner of a hospital room can suggest to one woman that things can go wrong, but to another may be reassuring. What you can see in a hospital may remind you of illness; if you see needles and have a needle phobia it may cause anxiety. At home, looking at a pile of washing or an untidy house may cause anxiety in some women. Seeing things around you that make you feel reassured, secure and familiar is very important.

Denis Walsh, Professor of Midwifery at Nottingham University, has written about how birthing rooms in hospital should be designed so that any medical equipment is kept out of sight and rooms are as homely as possible. This is being done to an extent in some hospitals where I've seen more homely furniture and soft lighting, with plenty of space to move around. Some units are now being purpose built to make a birthing unit a home from home, and even include double beds for after the birth.

Visual Anchor

To create a visual anchor think about taking something into your birth space that reminds you of a time when you were relaxed, or a time when you achieved something amazing. Perhaps you have something at home that reminds you of feeling confident and focused. One woman I taught had collected what she called her oxytocin photos. She took a set of photos into hospital that reminded her of events where she'd felt loving kindness, a sense of achievement and so on. Looking at these made her feel strong and capable.

What You Can Feel

Imagine that you are burying your head into your pillow, wrapped in your cosy duvet, with the warmth of your bed around you. You may be aware of your shoulders sinking at that thought. What we feel around us can contribute to a state of relaxation and comfort that is important for birth. Physical touch also brings a sense of comfort; some women don't like soft stroking during labour and may prefer a firmer touch of reassurance that has been anchored well using hypnosis.

Touch Anchor

Take your own pillow and a small blanket into your birth space. This will add a comforting familiarity to the room. The blanket can be thrown over the bed or around your shoulders to keep you warm after baby is born. These are ready-made anchors as you already associate them with feeling comfortable and secure.

You can also create a loving touch anchor with your birth partner. Put your hypnosis tracks on, and allow yourself to relax, then get your partner to rest their hand on your shoulder. Be aware of the reassuring, solid, supportive touch on your shoulder. Ask your partner to do this every five minutes when listening to the first hypnosis track, and find the time to do this once or twice a week. The more you do it, the stronger and more effective the anchor is. This will mean that every time your partner puts their hand on your shoulder you instantly feel confident, relaxed and calm.

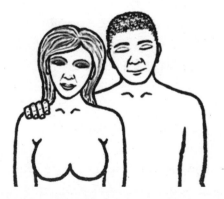

Practise this anchor. You can also put two hands on your partner's shoulders, one on each shoulder. This is a great technique, particularly if she needs a bit more support.

What You Can Hear

Hospitals are noisy places, with unfamiliar sounds all around. You may even be able to hear other women giving birth. The normal sounds of a hospital can be interruptions that bring a woman to a higher state of alert, quite literally listening out for danger. Careful consideration should be given to what you are likely to hear during labour in your chosen environment. It can work the other way too; at home some women are conscious of being overheard.

Your birth space should ideally be a quiet place where talk and chatter are kept to a minimum. While external noises are one thing to try and avoid, language is another thing to watch very carefully. Hypnotherapy is a therapy of language; hypnotherapists are always listening out for changes in language that betray deeper emotions and feelings. We also use language in a way that suggests change at an unconscious level. Language is powerful and how it is used, or not used, can change the course of a labour.

When we are in an endorphin-rich altered state of consciousness we become more suggestible; our thinking brain slows down and we accept suggestions and comments more easily than we would normally. This is why hypnosis is such a powerful therapy for change: it bypasses your conscious brain, your neo-cortex, changing things very quickly at a deeply unconscious level.

Gentle, soft-spoken suggestions, not requiring a response, can have a very positive effect: 'You're doing so well, everything is perfect, everything is as it should be.' If she has a strong contraction: 'That's right, fantastic, your body is doing so well. Each contraction is bringing your baby closer to us.' If she says she can't do it just whisper, 'In this moment you are doing it, just in this moment you can do it.'

I often see people trying to talk to a mum, loudly, in the middle of a contraction or when she is deeply focused, asking her what she wants, trying to establish rapport through language. Good rapport and reassurance can be just as powerful with a smile and a light hand on the shoulder or the upper arm.

Hearing Anchor

The background music on the hypnosis tracks is an anchor, as are the hypnosis tracks themselves. My voice becomes an anchor for many women. I once walked into a postnatal group and started talking to someone, when a woman I'd never met before said, 'It's you! Your voice makes me feel calm and relaxed even now; I listened to you all through my pregnancy and birth.'

Having headphones on can make a big difference as it can cut out background noise, as well as stopping people from starting up conversation with you. It's much easier to stay in your birthing zone when you cut out background noise as it's then that you can really go deep into hypnosis.

What You Can Smell

We don't always think about how dependent we may be on smell to orientate us in our lives. However, smell is one of the most effective ways to trigger responses as it's a form of 'chemoreception'. This means that our nose changes chemical signals straight into neural impulses, and our reaction to a smell is quicker than if we see or hear something. This is why hypnotic body conditioning using a smell is extremely fast-working and effective. Some environments harbour smells that can trigger a strong emotional and physical response. Hospitals are one of those, so the trick is to anchor a smell that overwhelms the hospital smell which so many people associate with illness.

Smell Anchor

Choose an aromatherapy oil that you like and which is safe to use during pregnancy. Lavender is a popular one. Then pop a bit nearby when you listen to your hypnosis tracks. You can put a couple of drops on your pillow, on a tissue tucked into your top, or you can use a diffuser which spreads the smell around the room. You could also have a diffuser at the birth. If you are using an oil burner and a flame, please be sure that you have it in a safe place; be aware that sometimes you may fall asleep after listening to the tracks. After practising this every day for a short while, not only will the smell relax you wherever you are but it will also cancel out any unwelcome smells in your birth environment. You can even get oil made up for you by an aromatherapist to be used as massage oil. Loving touch and a comforting smell is a great combination for loving birth, making you feel comfortable and supported.

WHO MAKES A BIRTH SPACE GREAT?

Who is with us is of course one of the most important things to get right. You will need someone loving and kind, supportive and, above all, patient. The qualities of your birthing partner should reflect the aspects discussed in Chapter 11, 'Turning a Birth Partner into a Hypnobirth Partner'.

In your midwives and doctors, you need health professionals that are patient, hands-off and trusting in birth. You'll need to be comfortable with your midwife; within minutes of meeting her you will get an instinctive sense of being comfortable or uncomfortable with her. If you don't like your midwife, don't feel guilty; do you get on with everyone you meet? You can always ask to change your midwife.

Having a partner, a friend or a doula, who can hold your space for you and stick to preferences, however birth is progressing or what length of time it's taking, is really important.

> **TIP:** A dad I was doula for came and spoke to my class and talked about how valuable it had been having someone else there. He suggested that if they can't have a doula for any reason, people find a friend they can call during the birth. This might be just for an hour here or there to give the partner time to collect themselves, get some fresh air, eat or even have a quick nap. Having rest breaks is important so that the birth partner feels refreshed and focused. Don't forget that the birth partner has a baby to look after as well after the birth.

I've seen women give birth surrounded by other women at home, and I've seen women on their own at home give birth suddenly while the midwife or the birthing partner is out of the room. You may find you don't want anyone there; you may find you want to be surrounded by family. Every woman is different. Make sure that you feel comfortable with who is in the room with you.

WHERE YOU CHOOSE TO BIRTH

Deciding whether to birth at hospital or home is very personal. Ideally, your midwife should give you a choice and impartial, evidence-based advice on the risks and benefits of a home birth and a hospital birth. It may be helpful to share your birth preferences with your midwife and ask her how the local hospital, midwife-led unit or community midwives would support those preferences based on your health and any previous pregnancies. She may be aware of how particular units or settings are more closely aligned with your preferences.

You may feel safer in hospital than at home. You may instinctively want to be at home but feel pressure to go into hospital; if so this pressure may come from other people and be rooted in their own fears and sense of responsibility. Your home can also be a factor in your choice. People who live nearly an hour away from the nearest hospital will probably want to birth in the hospital. Your home may be five minutes away so this could be less of a concern. There may also be neighbours to think about; you may be uncomfortable or worried about neighbours hearing you.

When you think of your birthing environment, you should feel relaxed; your gut instinct should tell you that you are in the right place. Don't let your decision come from a place of fear. Instead think, 'How can I make the birth space as familiar, comforting and welcoming as I possibly can? How can I make it my own?'

Which Environment is Right for me?

Considering all of the above, I've made a list of the benefits of each environment, as well as the negatives. It's up to you to decide, on balance, which is right for you. In my classes I do a short exercise on place of birth and hormones. Overwhelmingly, the men show that they are more relaxed in hospital where they feel secure and can hand responsibility over. On the other hand, women show that they are more oxytocin-rich at home because they are instinctively drawn to an environment where they feel familiar and in control.

Have a look through these tables which contain common responses in my classes. Then make your own so you can explore your reasons for being in hospital or at home with full awareness of the role of oxytocin.

Pros

Hospital Birth	Planned Home Birth
Medical help if my baby or I need it	Familiar environment
Access to more choices of pain relief	Intervention rates are lower
I can ask to change my midwife if I don't like her	You are in control, midwives are coming into your space
I get uninterrupted space with my baby if I have other children and I can restrict visitors	One-to-one care
I don't have to worry about an untidy house	Guaranteed your own pool
	Don't have to worry about 'going in at the right time'
	You can have as many birth partners as you want or as few, including other children if you wish
	Partner doesn't have to leave

Cons

Hospital Birth	Planned Home Birth
Unfamiliar environment	I or my baby may need medical care
Limited to two birth partners	I have to empty the pool
Midwife looking after other couples	Neighbours might hear me
Pool not guaranteed	I have other children
Intervention rates are higher	I may have to be transferred in an ambulance
Partner may have to go home after the birth	Limited choice of midwives
	I'm too far away from a hospital

A Home Birth

For many people, home is the natural environment for oxytocin. It is a familiar space; you are surrounded by your own smell, sounds and home comforts. You have freedom of movement, inviting people into your space rather than being invited into someone else's space.

There may be less unconscious pressure on you to progress. Community midwives may have more experience in undisturbed birth, and one-to-one care means that they are more able to watch for external changes in the mother that show how she is progressing through labour, rather than reaching for easily accessible equipment. All of this is favourable in how a mother reacts unconsciously, and therefore physically, to her environment during birth.

Is a Home Birth Safe?

In the UK the home birth rate is around 2.8 per cent, which is very low compared to countries such as Holland at around 29 per cent, but higher than the US which is around 0.7 per cent. One of the most important things when considering a home birth is dispelling the myth that birth is dangerous. If you are low risk, a home birth is a very real option. Even if you are not considered low risk, you can still research the evidence yourself and make an informed choice.

Several studies have been carried out into the safety of home birth compared to hospital birth. One of the most interesting is by a statistician called Marjory Tew, who didn't believe that home birth was safe; she meticulously catalogued and researched safety and birth settings. In her book *Safer Childbirth*, Tew showed why she had done a complete U-turn on her original thinking.

The Birthday Trust research, led by Professor Geoffrey Chamberlin, compared like-for-like mothers in an obstetric and home birth setting. It found that 'there was no evidence that women who had been screened properly in the antenatal period and who booked a planned delivery for home had any higher risk than a similar group of women who delivered in hospital'.

You may be surprised to discover that research published in the *British Medical Journal (BMJ)* in 2013 concluded that women 'were significantly less likely than those with planned births in obstetric units to have an instrumental or operative delivery or to receive medical interventions such as augmentation, epidural or spinal analgesia, general anaesthesia, or episiotomy and significantly more likely to have a "normal birth"'.

Home birth midwives are well trained to spot problems long before they become an issue. One midwife referred to it as watching a calm lake, and because you are aware and observing that lake, you become alert to a tiny ripple long before it becomes a tsunami. If your midwife sees a ripple, it may be nothing, but she will always err on the side of caution by suggesting a transfer to hospital. There is an assumption that if something goes wrong it happens instantly, but usually there are signs long before that midwives are trained and equipped to deal with.

A Hospital Birth

If you are low risk your birth should be in a midwifery-led unit, even in a hospital environment. These are typically more homely. If you are consultant led you may be in an obstetric-led unit where the rooms may be more clinical. In a hospital setting you do have options about your environment and can make changes that support a mindful hypnobirth, allowing you to let go and relax at both a conscious and unconscious level.

Whether you are high or low risk, these changes may include creating subdued lighting, putting on your own music, using your anchors (see page 111) and moving the bed to create space to move around. If you are in a midwifery-led unit, you may find that many of these things have already been put in place by the midwifery team. Once you are settled you can put your headphones on, use your breathing and get yourself centred in your birthing zone.

If you are on a monitor, simple things like switching the sound off or down and turning it away from your view can be really important. It's easy for both the mother and her partner to become fixated on a monitor, worrying about each dip or rise. Rather than helping a mother get into her birthing zone, the attention can turn to worry. I've been in a room with a monitor and they are hypnotic! A variable heart rate can be completely normal and the sign of a healthy, happy baby but to the untrained eye small dips can make you feel unsettled, all of which can slow down the release of oxytocin.

All the anchors that you have read about can be adapted to hospital, whether you are low or high risk. Rest assured that using hypnosis and mindfulness means that you are able to approach potential intervention in a positive frame of mind. If you are higher risk make the effort to learn about your choices and to talk to your consultant or midwife about keeping as closely to your birth preferences as you can.

If you are low risk and in a hospital setting, studies suggest that being midwifery led can improve outcomes. Compared with low-risk births attended by a doctor, midwife-attended low-risk births have less chance of problems with the birth and lead to less intervention.

It's not unusual for someone to start off being consultant led if they are considered higher risk, and if all continues normally to be transferred to the midwifery-led care. You can explore this option with your consultant closer to your birth and have it put on your notes if this is what you want. Even on the day you can ask to be moved to midwifery-led care, which may mean a more relaxed environment. I've seen women have relatively undisturbed births in very calm, dim and loving surroundings, including an induction, a mother with a baby that had to be very closely monitored and a mother with ME. When you feel comfortable and supported by those around you, it can give you the confidence to make choices that are right for you and your baby, wherever you choose to give birth.

Charlotte's waters broke before labour started and had meconium in them, which can be normal but can also be a sign that baby is compromised. Charlotte's antenatal care had been with an independent midwife. She recommended that they go into hospital for monitoring and to check that all was fine. I met Charlotte at the hospital and they popped her on a monitor to check baby was well. We had a wonderful, patient midwife who talked Charlotte through what she was doing, and spent some time fixing 'long leads' to the monitor so that Charlotte could move around and get off the bed. We moved the bed to the side with her help, tucked the monitor in the corner away from Charlotte and her partner, with the sound turned off. The lights were turned down, a birthing ball brought in, and the midwife made up a calming mix of aromatherapy oils that were massaged into Charlotte's bump. (If an induction is suggested, you may be waiting around and there is plenty of time to do all this.) The doctor wanted to induce Charlotte to get things moving and advised an oxytocin drip. However, we went through other choices, which were to leave her on the monitor and wait for things to start normally, to have a pessary, or to have the drip. The midwife talked through all her options and Charlotte chose to have the drip. During the course of labour a doctor came in and sat with Charlotte because he had never seen an induction that was so relaxed; he could see she was having contractions on the monitor but she was talking to him with little awareness of them. As the drip was turned up and the contractions got stronger, Charlotte held her anchor, which was a soft knitted heart with lavender oil on it, and breathed through each contraction with the support of her partner. She got on and off the bed, so movement and massage were important. Her contractions did get very intense but she got into a great rhythm and her little girl was born without any other intervention.

SUMMARY

- Wherever you choose to birth, think about preparing to make the environment as comfortable as you can. Anchors are triggers that give the body the signal to relax and let go, sending the message that you feel secure, with a sense of familiarity around you.
- Prepare your anchors so you can alter your environment quickly at the birth.
- Think about your senses and things that make you feel confident, relaxed and calm.

11

TURNING A BIRTH PARTNER INTO A HYPNOBIRTH PARTNER

Speak tenderly to them. Let there be kindness in your face, in your eyes, in your smile. Always have a cheerful smile. Don't only give your care, but give your heart as well.

Mother Teresa

This section is written for your birth partner.

Your role as birth partner is such an important one. You will be the emotional and physical support for your partner as she brings your baby into the world. You may have prepared by reading or going to antenatal classes, or perhaps you feel under prepared. Mindful hypnobirthing preparation focuses more on emotional preparation and how you can learn to be a strong and centred partner, free of your own judgment and fears around birth.

SHOULD A MAN BE AT THE BIRTH?

Until the last century, women would be near their mothers, sisters and aunts when they gave birth. As we've developed economically and become more industrialised, people have moved to cities where jobs were away from their traditional family units. This means that in today's society a birth partner is more likely to be a life partner, rather than their mother or other women in the family or community. It is important for a woman to feel safe and protected during labour. Research shows that – consistent with tradition – a trusted female, independent from the family, gives consistently better birth outcomes, but in the absence of this a well-prepared birth partner can be just as good.

Men who are in attendance at their baby's birth and hold their baby shortly afterwards have very similar feelings of attachment to those experienced by mothers for the first two weeks. This experience is shown also to have a longer-term impact, with fathers who attended the birth being more involved in their children as they grow up. Having a father who is engaged, emotionally invested and connected in his children's lives can only be of benefit to the child, the mother and the family unit.

In my view, a good birth partner – irrespective of whether it's a man or a woman – is worth their weight in gold. As long as you are both comfortable, you know what your role is and can let go of the need to control the space based on your own needs, you can be the best possible support. When you trust your partner completely, when you care for her during her labour with loving kindness, compassion and strength, you will be the vessel that helps carry her and your baby on their birth journey.

DADS HAVE CHOICES TOO

Overwhelmingly, people talk about mothers exerting their choices and being in control of their birth but very rarely do we speak of the father's wishes. If you do not want to be at the birth, or certain aspects of birth make you feel uncomfortable, it will make a difference to the birth. You'll more than likely release adrenaline, which is contagious, and can affect how the mother feels and how her body responds to labour. If you don't want to actually see baby coming out – and this is not unusual in my experience as a doula – this should be respected. If you don't want to cut the cord this too should be respected. I've seen overzealous midwives insist the dad see the baby being born, and reluctant dads dragged down to cut the cord. Your needs have to be respected as well.

If for some reason the mother doesn't want you there, don't take it as an affront. Some women don't feel comfortable really letting go in front of their partner. I've known women to give birth when their husband has nipped out to get a coffee.

PREPARING EMOTIONALLY

To prepare emotionally, it's important to spend time reflecting on your baby and your partner's pregnancy. Take time out for the two of you to talk about your baby, but also to talk *to* your baby. I know many men do this instinctively; they may read the football score out to their baby, sing or play music to their baby. Although a baby doesn't necessarily hear sounds in the same way as we do, they are aware of very subtle differences in cadence, the rhythm of language, that are unique to each individual. Certain rhythms are soothing to babies; research shows babies are very aware of rhythm and can recall certain strains of music, from soap opera theme tunes through to baroque, so the rhythm of the father's voice is very familiar and comforting. Babies turn their head or move towards the direction of their father's voice. A baby who has heard him speaking directly to them regularly will recognise their father's voice and feel calmer when that voice is nearby, even after they are born. When my first son was born, I watched amazed as he turned his eyes to where my husband's voice was on the other side of the room, clearly seeking him out.

Making that connection with your baby on a regular basis, and acknowledging them as a part of your family while in the womb, will also allow you to slowly adjust and get used to having another person in your relationship. Make sure that you spend time doing some of the exercises in this book with your partner as well so you can build a connection with her and the baby, and learn how to help support her in these techniques.

Make Time for Antenatal Appointments

Talk to your partner about her antenatal appointments and take some time off to go to these appointments with her, even if they are routine. Although there is no legal right for men to have time off for antenatal appointments in the UK, the Government recommends that employers allow fathers either to take paid time off, or to make up the time later. Having the opportunity to listen to your baby's heartbeat on a regular basis and being part of those appointments can be a simple but profound way to connect emotionally with your baby.

There are many books with practical advice on helping a partner prepare for a birth, some of which I have listed in the Resources section (see page 232). What I want to get you to think about in this book is the emotional support that is needed at a birth and for you to explore your own fears and worries. You'll also learn a few additional practical things to do in the room that can help a hypnobirth.

THREE DIFFERENT ROLES, IN ONE

If you've attended NHS or NCT classes you may have an idea of what to expect at the birth. However, if you're doing hypnobirthing or preparing mindfully, the approach to take will be slightly different. There are three roles for the birthing partner:

- The Practical Partner
- The Protective Partner
- The Mindful Partner

These three roles clearly define the different aspects of a birthing partner's job, which all contribute to allowing mum to switch off and trust that everything is taken care of. The detail of these three jobs will be unique for each individual couple, so it's up to you to sit down and go through the things that are important for you.

The Practical Partner

This role is about, yes you've guessed it, the practical jobs. It's really important that you're not asking your partner where everything is or how things need to be when she's going within herself during labour. Some practical jobs may be fairly obvious, such as making sure that the bag is in the car, that you have money for parking and so forth. Others may take a little more thought, like getting the room right according to what you've learned in this book. The practical element also includes the more hands-on activity such as massage and physical touch.

> **TIP:** Find a class or book a session with a massage therapist who specialises in birth so you can learn some hands-on massage techniques for during the birth. These can be comforting and help release oxytocin.

The Practical Partner Checklist

- ☐ Lights off in the room
- ☐ Aromatherapy oil
- ☐ Blanket/bedroom pillow on the bed
- ☐ Hypnosis tracks on CD and MP3 player, headphones
- ☐ Affirmations
- ☐ Money
- ☐ Food and drink stocks
- ☐ Warm wheat bag or cool cloths

The Protective Partner

Sometimes I think that this is the hardest role. I used to feel that using the word 'gatekeeper' was adversarial, divisive and anti-medical. A midwife I knew and respected changed my mind. If a woman is coming into hospital she may have to pass through four or five gates herself that belong to someone else. There's the entrance to the hospital, the reception, the doors to the labour suite, then maybe another set of doors to the midwifery- or consultancy-led unit and then the room itself. This midwife understood that the mother would be in an unfamiliar environment. It's absolutely her right to have someone acting as a gatekeeper for her, so that she feels safe and that someone she trusts is looking out for her.

Being the gatekeeper is also important when your partner is in her birthing zone, deep in labour. The aim is to keep her in that state by slowing down neo-cortical activity. Questions from medical staff and conversations with the mother all activate her neo-cortex. If the room has been dark and someone switches a light on, it can jolt her from her birthing zone; or if several people bustle into the room it can imbue a sense of being watched, activating her alert systems and 'waking' her up.

The job of the gatekeeper is to make sure that the birth preferences are respected. If the birth preferences say 'Could you speak to my partner before interrupting me?' then the staff should speak to you first. If the birth preferences read 'Please do not offer me pain relief, I'll ask for it if I need it', they shouldn't offer her it, and it's your job to make sure that this is adhered to.

Communication

A good birthing partner will be able to talk to the midwives or the doctors before the mother needs to be consulted and buy more time, or decline an intervention based on the birth preferences and discussions the couple has had before the birth. The difficulty many people have is allowing themselves to think, 'I'm not a doctor or a midwife, I don't have medical training, how can I make these choices?' It can be difficult but you don't have to be a medical expert to make decisions; you just need to have enough of the benefits and risks explained to you in order to make an informed choice.

In Chapter 8, I discussed the BRAINS questions (see page 97). This is given out in many antenatal classes across the country and is a very clearly defined set of questions that enable you to get the information you need to make a choice. If labour has slowed down and they want to speed it up, the question to ask is, 'Is mum fine and is the baby fine?' If the answer is 'yes', then question why that intervention is needed. Always remember that the philosophy of normal birth is uninterrupted birth. Yes, birth can sometimes take a while and it can be unpredictable, so it's important to have patience. If all is well, ask yourself why you need this intervention. You may be told several *potential* things that could go wrong, especially if the medical team is advising you to have a particular intervention, but remind yourself that in this moment all is well. In this way you can bide your time, and keep that space free of anxiety or worry for the mother. Rest assured that if something were to go wrong the medical team would react very, very quickly.

The other job of the gatekeeper is to build up a relationship with your midwife. If you are in a situation where you are trying to assert the wishes of the mother, it's not uncommon for midwives to feel uncomfortable: they are used to talking to the mother, and are trained to build up rapport with her. This is where unconscious communication can cause some difficulties. If the midwife is distracted, dismissive or not really listening to the wishes of the couple it can create a sense of unease. In a busy hospital unit, where she may be caring for several couples, it takes skill and empathy to be able to switch off from one couple and to really *be* with another couple a few minutes later. A birthing partner feels an instinct to protect his partner. When this happens, body language changes; we may release adrenaline and appear more aggressive; this in turn makes the midwife perhaps feel uncomfortable and then see the couple as demanding and uncooperative.

Being a Compassionate Communicator

Engaging with the midwife with compassion, perhaps asking for her assistance and experience in helping you stay as close to your birth preferences as possible, can make a huge difference. I've found just lowering my voice and slowing my breathing down can help; as does changing my body language so that my arms are by my side and my shoulders are down.

Make sure that your body language says 'I am open to your views and I care about what you have to say to me'. Tilt your head slightly to one side, which tells her unconsciously that you are listening to her. If she says she's busy, use what is known as reflective language: 'I understand that you are busy, when you are ready …' Midwives aren't superhuman, though sometimes they seem to be; they are human beings under pressure who respond to acknowledgment and empathy too. She may be newly qualified and frightened about doing something that she hasn't learned about; she may be under the weather; she may be distracted by an emergency in another room.

This is why I think being a gatekeeper can be so hard. This is your day, one of the biggest days of your life. Your child is being born – surely you deserve 100 per cent attention and the midwife should be there for you when you need her? The truth is that hospitals are understaffed and midwives are under pressure in their jobs, which affects how they are able to care for you. If you have a home birth there is likely to be much less pressure to accept intervention, and with one-to-one care it's much easier to build up a relationship with the midwife, who may also be more relaxed and comfortable in your home.

The Protective Partner Checklist
- ❏ BRAINS sheet from page 97
- ❏ Practise the exercise 'Three, two, one, relax, relax, relax' (see page 46)
- ❏ Three copies of your birth preferences
- ❏ Any research that supports choices important to you

The Mindful Partner

All the practical and proactive support that a birthing partner gives is important for getting the environment absolutely right. This allows the mother to let go completely, free of worry or anxiety. When a mother is in labour, she may not wish to talk or converse. If she's using hypnobirthing she will be in her birthing zone. You may know when she's having a contraction or you may not be aware at all. I've been with women who are very obviously having a contraction and make as much noise as they can, and others who I could only tell from the curl of their toe or a hiccup afterwards.

Being in the birthing zone doesn't necessarily mean that she will be completely silent and not ask questions or speak with you.

I've been with mothers who were very deeply focused during contractions and irritated by interruption or lights coming on and I've been with mothers who were making noise. Some women are able to make conversation between contractions, and others may appear to ask questions without expecting an answer. The instinct of a partner is to answer those questions directly. However, after watching many women, I realised that when women in labour begin to ask questions that seem unfocused or don't quite make sense they are largely rhetorical: they don't need an answer. In fact, an answer can begin a conversation that can start to lift her out of that altered state. When I work in a therapeutic environment, people who are processing an emotion or an experience may express it in the form of a rhetorical question, not expecting an answer from me but instead seeking that answer from within themselves. I've seen the same process happen frequently at births.

Birth Talk, Sleep Talk

When women are deep in their birthing zone, if they speak it can be a little like sleep talking. I first experienced this with one of my doula clients who was going through transition. She was getting agitated and upset, shaking her head and saying, 'I can't do this any more, I need an epidural.' She'd been fine up until then, so a knowing nod and smile from the midwife reassured us that she was in transition.

Instead of trying to find things that would make it better for her by asking her what she wanted or making suggestions, when she wandered over to me I just took her head in my hands, looked her in the eyes and with a smile and a firm voice said, 'You think you can't do this, but you can. We are with you, you are strong.' Her pupils were dilated, and she said in a dreamy voice, 'Yes, yes I can, I can,' then turned and wandered away from me, swaying gently. It was at that moment that I knew many questions should be reflected back, or treated as rhetorical. In most instances a simple positive suggestion that doesn't require a response will do. Even non-verbal responses can be very powerful. If you were to look into your partner's eyes, hold her hands and give a reassuring smile after each contraction or when she opened her eyes it would send a very powerful message that 'all is well, you're doing great, I love you and I am here for you'.

> **TIP:** Try reflecting what she is saying. If she says, 'I can't do this any more,' say, 'I know you think that, you can do it, I am here for you.' You are acknowledging her fear, but also using very subtle hypnotic suggestion. Read it out loud and see how it sounds.

Being Present

Just a strong, quiet presence can make all the difference. Birth can be quick and it can take time but knowing there is someone there looking out for you and watching out for danger can reduce the levels of adrenaline and nor-adrenaline in the mother, allowing labour to progress. Sometimes this means just sitting there quietly and being in that moment, either awake or asleep in the chair next to her.

My mother's friends reminded me that when midwives provided one-to-one care at home, they would sit in the chair and knit; the sound of knitting needles was associated with the midwives. Knitting meant that the midwife was there, quietly observing but not watching; this is an important distinction. I've sat in a chair for 12 hours with short breaks and just massaged a mother's leg, while no word was uttered or eye opened. It was like sitting watching someone sleep. Just because she didn't communicate with her partner or me didn't mean our presence wasn't valued. After the birth she said that in her head she knew when one of us left the room and when I neglected to massage her foot during a contraction!

To be a mindful partner you can prepare yourself using some of the hypnosis techniques in Part Two of this book. You could also try the following exercise. Alternatively, you can take something with you, such as a book, crosswords or sudokus. Be aware, though, that mothers have commented negatively on their partners being on phones or computers.

This short exercise is sometimes used as an induction for hypnosis but is also a very effective mindfulness exercise that I use when I'm at a birth, perhaps in the middle of the night, or when I start to feel myself becoming more alert and tense at a birth.

The Four Awarenesses

Sit quietly in a chair, looking straight ahead and roll your eyes back as far as is just about comfortable. Find something to fix your eyes on, such as a spot on the ceiling, a light or a shadow. Without moving your head or your eyes, you are going to think of four things you can see, four things you can feel and four things you can hear, then three things you can see, feel and hear, two things you can see, feel and hear and then one. If at any moment your eyes feel tired just shut them and continue to feel and hear in no particular order.

'I can see the light, I can see movement, I can see the curtain, I can see the picture, I can hear traffic, I can hear my breathing, I can hear the washing machine, I can hear a voice, I can feel my weight on the chair, I can feel my stomach rumbling, I feel tired, I feel the warmth of my hand on my leg, I can see light, I can see movement, I can see the picture, I can hear traffic, I can hear …' and so on.

> Sometimes you may lose track; that's fine, go with it
> and with what comes to mind in that moment. I sometimes
> find that I settle on a sound or a feeling as I close my eyes,
> usually the sound of the traffic or the feel of my breath.

I'M AFRAID OF SEEING MY PARTNER IN PAIN

It's natural for a man to want to protect and care for his partner.
For some men the hardest thing can be seeing the woman he loves
experience such physical intensity and not know how to help. A
man's instinct may be to want to rescue her from that situation.
Seeing the person they love act out of character may also make
him feel very uncomfortable. This is usually one of the biggest
concerns of men who come to my classes.

Birth is a very intense experience. The woman may not be
suffering, although your own perception may be that she is. A
partner's reactions are based on preconceptions and assumptions
about birth derived from what they've been told second hand or
have seen on television.

*If you are privileged enough to have witnessed a woman giving
birth unaided in a place she has chosen, what will you have
seen? You will first be in awe of her strength. Her thighs stand
strong and mighty like those of a warrior as she stands, sways
and squats to find the best position to ease her baby out. Then
you will hear the deep primal cries she makes as she does her
work, sounds that come not from her throat but from her belly
as she grunts and moans with her exertion: sounds seldom heard
except in the most uninhibited of love-making. Maybe you will
notice the glistening river of mucus tinged with blood and waters
that run down her thighs unheeded: she is beyond noticing such*

things, moved as she has done into another plane of existence. And then finally you will be struck by her beauty: her face softened with the flow of oxytocin, her eyes wide and shining, her pupils dark, deep and open. And you will think — for how could you not — what a phenomenal creature is a woman. But you will only have seen this astonishing sight if you understand that if you disturb her in her work, she will be thrown off course. Like a zoologist, you must first learn how to behave; how to sit quietly and patiently, almost invisible, breathing with her, not disturbing her mighty internal rhythm. And you will see that the pain of her labours seldom overwhelms her. Nature would not have organised labour to be intolerable.

(Leap and Anderson 2004: 28)

What if I Start Feeling Anxious?

If your partner's instinct is to make noise, and to express herself in a more extroverted way, you might not know how to deal with this. Your first thought may be to offer pain relief, even if the mother has said she doesn't want it, or it may be to assume that something is wrong and begin to worry. The assumption that something is wrong can trigger a release of adrenaline in the father, which may in turn be picked up by the mother at an unconscious level. If

> **TIP:** If you start feeling anxious or impatient, ask for the midwife to sit with your partner while you go and get some air. Leave the room, maybe go and get a cup of tea or something to eat. Just sit quietly and centre yourself until you feel that anxiety dropping. Then when you are ready you can return to the room. You will be a much better birth partner for that.

this happens it's incredibly important that you are able to observe that feeling arising within you and allow her the space to express herself in the way that she feels she wants to: free of judgment.

As labour progresses, her contractions may get stronger and longer. They may seem closer together; at some point they may even seem as if they are coming on top of each other. Your partner may say she can't do this any more, even if she has been coping well up to this point. She may demand an epidural and be very determined to get one. It's very likely that this is a stage called transition (see page 186). Midwives can very quickly spot a woman in transition, as there is a naturally occurring surge of adrenaline at a specific point in labour, and even women who have been breathing in a very focused way can suddenly change.

For the birth partner this can be a challenge, but it's important that at this point your partner uses some of the techniques you will have learned in preparing for a hypnobirth. You can be

---

TIPS FOR A BIRTH PARTNER:

1. Stay calm. Use breathing techniques yourself if you feel anxious.
2. Remember to use the affirmations for the birth partner on page 76–77.
3. Don't feel the need to start up conversation.
4. Be strong and confident – she will feel this.
5. Trust that all is well. If the midwife is concerned she will tell you.
6. If your partner says she is scared, acknowledge her fear: 'I understand you are scared, I love you and I am here for you.'

there emotionally for your partner by making use of many of the techniques. You can practise these with your partner, who will benefit by being able to stay centred, relaxed and calm.

SUMMARY

- By sitting there quietly and calmly you are being a great hypnobirth partner.
- Think about your different roles.
- Learn to be accepting of the process and trust that she can do this.
- If she wants anything she will ask for it.
- Most of all be strong, supportive, loving, gentle, patient and kind.

12

WHEN WILL I GO INTO LABOUR?

One of the most important things I have learned about birthing babies is that the process is more of an unfolding marvel than a routine progression of events.

Tori Kropp

While you are practising your hypnosis techniques every day, preparing your mind for birth, your body is preparing quietly for your baby's birth. You are not aware of many of these intricate changes in your body as hormones trigger adjustments that are perfectly attuned to your body and your baby. It can be really helpful to know what your hormones are doing and to bring awareness to physical changes that can guide you and inform you of how things are changing in preparation for labour.

THE FINAL WEEKS OF PREGNANCY

Each woman births in her 'uniquely normal' way, just as you will. Being mindful of the interconnectivity of the hormonal balance between your body, your baby and your brain can help you build your confidence in how you birth, whichever path it takes. Each individual woman has a unique sensitivity to her own hormones, and her balance is perfect for her.

Your Hormones Are on the Move

Your hormones are busy preparing your body for conception, pregnancy and birth while you are going about your daily life. If you knew how busy your body was you'd be amazed! It's a bit like King's Cross Station: hormones on the move, travelling around going to different places, all in preparation for the birth of your baby. Their journeys, arrivals and departures are all dependent on train times. Sometimes the trains run a little late; maybe they are on a slow cross-country route. Think of your brain preparing and coordinating all those different journeys; it's quite a complicated task but it does it just fine. The best thing is to just let it get on with it.

You are your hormones: the exchange of those hormones is so unique, so precise and so delicate that it's impossible to adjust or accurately interfere with it. Imagine a clock with a very intricate movement, each part designed to hold the other so it works harmoniously to bring you the perfect time. Understanding how familiar changes during pregnancy are triggered by hormonal shifts can really help you see how capable your body is of going into labour and managing it in the best and most comfortable way for you and your baby.

HOW YOUR HORMONES SHIFT FROM PREGNANCY TO BIRTH

Relaxin

In the weeks before labour, the body releases relaxin, which is produced by the corpus luteum, breasts and placenta. Relaxin reaches peaks at around 14 weeks of pregnancy and when your baby is due to be born. Signs of relaxin are sometimes heartburn and discomfort in the pelvis. Relaxin's job is to increase the space baby has to pass through the birth canal by softening the ligaments in your pelvis. Relaxin also softens the cervix in preparation for birth, sometimes a few weeks before your baby is born. Recent research also suggests that relaxin is the hormone responsible for vaso-dilation, which helps dilate blood vessels and decrease blood pressure. This is important as your blood volume increases by around 40–50 per cent during pregnancy to accommodate changes in your body and regulate nourishment for your baby.

Progesterone

The hormone progesterone rises during pregnancy, helping soften muscles in the womb for growth. It also helps protect the placenta by fighting off unwanted cells, and strengthens the mucosal lining, part of which you might know better as the mucus plug, which helps stop infection from entering the womb. Progesterone begins to taper off before birth, which is a signal to oestrogen to increase. Oestrogen and progesterone work closely together. Progesterone is an important hormone in conception and during pregnancy, as it helps the lining of the womb grow and prevents menstruation. It also helps improve nutrition for the baby, and works in synergy with oestrogen to prepare for breastfeeding. Early in pregnancy, there are high levels of the hormone hCG, which helps ensure high progesterone levels continue to be released by the corpus luteum before the placenta takes over progesterone production. The corpus luteum is like a mini hormone exchange located in your ovary that temporarily supports and maintains an environment for pregnancy to establish, before the placenta can develop and take over. Our body responds to these hormone changes with common pregnancy indicators such as sickness, headaches, food cravings, tiredness and breast tenderness. Towards the third and fourth month, hCG begins to drop once progesterone is released from the placenta and these symptoms begin to subside.

Oestrogen

Oestrogen is a very important hormone during pregnancy: it's responsible for the growth of the uterus, your breasts and breast ducts, which in turn help with producing milk and preparing you for breastfeeding. It also increases the capacity for contractions by upping the number of oxytocin receptors and 'gap junctions' in your womb lining and around your cervix. These gap junctions are incredibly important; they are the communication centres during labour and are like a telephone exchange between all the different hormones, helping regulate contractions and soften and open your cervix.

Your Hormones as You Prepare for Birth

Levels of oestrogen and progesterone both increase during pregnancy, but progesterone begins to taper off in the seventh month while oestrogen continues to rise. This is in readiness for labour when an increased ratio of oestrogen means that your womb is able to soften, expand and contract more efficiently. It's remarkable that the hormones in your body reverse their function through those communication centres set up during pregnancy. The hormones that have helped keep your cervix closed and your baby safe in the nine months they've been in your womb, begin to decrease and the ones that help the tissues in your body soften in preparation for birth increase.

To encourage labour to start, as progesterone tapers off, the increasing oestrogen released from the placenta triggers the release of prostaglandins. Prostaglandins are messengers in the tissues around your cervix that relay messages between your cervix, womb and brain to help trigger labour. Sometimes if you are over your dates your midwife will offer you a sweep. This is when she will sweep her fingers around your cervix and amniotic sack to try and trigger labour. If you have chosen to have a sweep, you are likely to be very near birth and these hormonal exchanges will already be in motion as they begin days and sometimes weeks before labour starts. So when the midwife says to you, 'Your cervix is soft and thin,' this means your body's hormones have already started preparing for labour.

Your mucus plug is a jelly-like substance that acts as a seal during pregnancy and is held by your cervix, which is closed. Another sign that your hormones are getting your body ready for the birth of your baby is the loss of some of your mucus plug, otherwise known as your 'show'. As your cervix softens and thins, the plug loosens and parts of it can fall away. You may notice it, or you may not; it may just be like clear thick vaginal discharge or it may be thick and streaked with a bit of blood. This is normal and can happen weeks, days or hours before labour starts, but it always means that your body's hormones are getting you and your baby ready for birth.

Imagine that your fist, like your cervix, is closed tight and you have some egg white in it, then imagine gently and slowly opening your fist. Some of the egg white will fall away, but not all until your fist is fully open.

WHAT TRIGGERS LABOUR?

A complex exchange of hormones between your baby and your body triggers labour and is timed in a way that is unique to you and your baby. Until recently, it was thought that the baby sets off this chain of events. However, research shows that labour may be triggered at the point when the energy demands of your baby are beginning to increase beyond that which your body can support.

Only then will your baby prepare to be born by increasing levels of what are known as androgens and releasing cortisol, which help your baby mature their lungs and prepare for life outside the womb.

When baby's lungs have received this boost, this in turn sets off hormonal changes in you, which will start labour. You may be aware of an increase in prostaglandins because it also triggers loose stools or diarrhoea, a common sign that labour is about to start. This means that the area around your uterus and bowels is softening, opening and relaxing in preparation for baby being born. I always ask my doula clients to text me if they get diarrhoea or loose bowels around their due date! You may be surprised to hear that fewer than 60 per cent of women experience contractions as the start of their labour, and instead recognise waters breaking, loose stools, blood staining, emotional changes or sleep alterations as a sign that labour has started.

Prostaglandins, unlike other hormones, are not produced in the brain, but are messengers located in tissue all around the body. They are present in high numbers around the tissue of the cervix, and prepare the cervix to open. As the cervix opens and softens, the stretching and pressure from your baby's head triggers the oxytocin receptors to leap into action and stimulate the release of oyxtocin.

The release of oxytocin triggers contractions, which in turn trigger more oxytocin to be released, triggering more contractions. This is the positive feedback loop. Early contractions during labour may be felt more in the lower area of your uterus, while your cervix is softening and thinning in response to the prostaglandins and low levels of oxytocin. Sometimes they are described by women as tweaks and niggles and are a positive sign that your body is getting its act together and starting to stretch and expand, coordinating its needs for labour. As labour becomes more established, oxytocin rises and contractions get closer together. Now a pressure or tightening may be felt more across the top half, or fundal area, of your uterus.

WHAT CAN I DO TO SUPPORT MY BODY?

The first thing you can do is to listen to your body. Recognise these changes and shifts in your body as steps towards labour, each small change a step on the path of your birth journey. Allow yourself to enjoy the view. Slow down; don't hurry to get to your destination; let yourself be carried along by your body as your legs would carry you on a walk or a run. Be confident that you will reach your destination.

Nurture your Body

Nurture your body as you would nurture your baby. Eating healthily will help your body get into the optimum state for birth. Studies show that some complications such as pre-eclampsia – a serious complication that affects mother and baby – may be connected to diet. When you are in a good frame of mind you will find that you gravitate naturally to more healthy food. Some women don't eat properly when they are anxious and worried; they either don't eat enough or eat too much of the wrong things, comfort foods. Make sure that your diet is healthy and rich with vegetables. Listen to what your body does and doesn't want to eat.

If you exercise, don't stop because you are pregnant; carry on with what you normally do. Keeping fit and healthy is important and will help you after your baby is born as well. Classes such as pregnancy yoga and Pilates are increasingly popular for preparing for labour; many mums I have worked with find they complement the hypnosis and mindfulness techniques very well.

Nurture your Mind

At around 37 weeks you should increase your mindful hypnobirth practice and be doing it every day, even if you have struggled to fit it in before. Consider stopping work earlier. You may be thinking that by working right up to the last minute you are buying time afterwards, yet those weeks before your baby is born are so important as they give you time to adjust and adapt to a slower pace of life. Sometimes, stopping a busy job, going into labour and caring for a baby in the space of what can be days can be an emotional roller-coaster, even without the hormonal shifts! Be kind to yourself and your hormones. Find a balance before your baby is born, and enjoy those last few quiet weeks of pregnancy by relaxing and centring yourself before labour begins and you become a mother.

SUMMARY

- In your final weeks of pregnancy, allow yourself to slow down.
- Make sure that you are practising your techniques daily.
- Tune in to your body.
- See changes as positive indications that your body is warming up for labour in its own perfect way.

PART 2
BIRTH

13

THIS IS IT! SIGNS THAT LABOUR HAS STARTED

300,000 women will be giving birth with you today. Relax and breathe and do nothing else … it's hard work, but you can do it.

Anon

For a first-time mum, looking out for signs that labour has started can be very confusing. Labour doesn't just start; it is a gradual series of changes and shifts in your body until you notice them enough to think you are in labour. These are often hormonal changes marked by physical changes, such as your plug coming away, loose stools, niggles in your lower uterus, awareness of baby being very low, perhaps even a very good night's sleep! Nature is kind like that.

I sometimes say to dads, if their partner seems a little spaced out and more absent-minded than usual, it may be a sign that oxytocin is building, and she is beginning to get into her birthing zone. Being able to recognise the signs that your body is warming up can be helpful as can knowing when is the right time to call the midwife or go to hospital.

HOW WILL I KNOW LABOUR HAS BEGUN?

If you have had a baby before, you are likely to be much more relaxed about labour starting. When labour starts for one person may be completely different for another. The clinical way of assessing whether you are in established labour is when you are 4–5 cm dilated. However, you may feel you are in labour before, or even after, this.

One of the most common mistakes first-time mums make is thinking that they should go to hospital as soon as something starts to happen. If you do go into hospital too early, this may lead to what is known as augmentation – help to speed labour up or get it started again. If this happens it may sometimes be that labour hasn't really got into its rhythm and is just warming up. This very subjective perspective of when labour has started may also be one of the reasons why second-time mums have much quicker labours.

Claire was due to have her second baby. Her first birth had been a 15-hour labour. She rang the hospital straight away when feeling strong contractions every four to five minutes and was told to come in. She was 4 cm dilated on admittance. At around 1pm she was told her baby was still high and contractions had slowed; if her waters were broken it would speed things up again. Once her waters had been broken, her labour got more intense so she had an epidural and was on the bed with a monitor. Around five hours later her baby was born with help from forceps.

Her second labour followed a similar pattern but she saw it a very different way.

In the morning she thought something was happening. She was getting lots of what she called 'niggles', which she thought were quite regular but then they faded away. She admitted she was distracted by her two year old. At around 3pm, I got a text saying she was getting childcare 'just in case'. At 7pm, I had a text to say that things were definitely beginning, and at 10pm she asked me to come over. When I arrived she was on the floor rocking on her hands and knees with her hypnosis track on in the background. She was talking between contractions and then going into her breathing during them. Although they were five minutes apart, she felt it wasn't the right time. Then suddenly she knew it was different and we headed off to the hospital. When we got up to the unit for assessment she was 8 cm dilated and 30 minutes later her waters broke. An hour after that her baby was born.

BRAXTON HICKS AND WARMING UP

Braxton Hicks contractions are often referred to as warm-up contractions as that's just what they are. Your body is warming up for labour. They can be a painless tightening or sometimes you will need to really focus on your breathing. They can start weeks before labour or in the days before.

Not everyone gets Braxton Hicks but they can sometimes feel like the real thing, tricking you into thinking labour has started. They may be regular and last for a few hours then just fade away, perhaps starting up again later that day or even the next. If this happens to you, imagine it as your body just finding its rhythm. I sometimes say to mums that these contractions can be like turning an engine over: you may need to turn it over a couple of times before the engine catches and starts.

Use these early warm-up contractions to practise your techniques, taking opportunities to rest in between. Maybe have a shower or a bath if they are quite strong. Perhaps go out for a walk, or just carry on with your daily life. Second-time mums often don't notice these contractions because they are distracted with other things, especially the care of other children, whereas a first-time mum tends to look out for every sign, amplifying what is really happening.

My Baby is Engaging. What Does this Mean?

You may be told by your midwife that your baby is engaging. This means that your baby is beginning to drop down into the pelvis ready for labour. This can happen weeks or days before, or – especially if you've had children before – right at the last minute, sometimes in labour itself. You may experience your baby engaging as a feeling of baby being very low; some women say that they feel their baby is about to fall out. They won't! It may feel as if you have niggles and that your baby is scrabbling around, but remember if your baby is engaged it means that their head is fitted into your pelvis and movement is more restricted for them.

TUNING IN TO THE RHYTHM OF LABOUR

Braxton Hicks contractions may be mistaken as early labour by first-time mums. Trust that you'll know when you are in labour and when your contractions get stronger and longer. Some women may have contractions five minutes apart for the whole of their labour; others will start at ten, go to seven minutes apart, then gradually to three minutes apart. A midwife might say, 'Are there three in ten or four in ten?', meaning are there three contractions in ten minutes or four contractions in ten minutes.

The niggles in your uterus begin to form a more distinct pattern and move upwards into your abdomen. Your abdomen will tighten with each contraction, pushing your baby's head on to your cervix.

It's like a tight hug for your baby. Each time your baby's head pushes down on your cervix, your cervix opens a little more.

> Take a little ball of play dough and roll it into a thick roll about 3 cm long and 3 cm wide. Now make a fist and gently roll it on the end of the play dough, putting gentle pressure on it as you do it. Continue to do this as the play dough begins to shorten and widen. Keep doing it until a small hole begins to appear in the middle of the playdough. Your baby's head is like your fist putting gentle pressure on your cervix, softening it and opening it.

This is why position is so important, and movement in early labour can certainly help to jiggle baby around so they get into the perfect position. When your baby is in a good position, it means that the head is fitted snugly on the cervix, allowing it open softly and quickly. As labour gets more established, you can begin to use your techniques; however, you may still be able to continue to do other things when the contractions are quite far apart. Too many women stop everything and focus in on the contractions when they are still quite far apart and lasting under a minute. Remember what you learned about focus, and how when you focus on something you can amplify it.

There is a short film by a midwife called 'The Birthday' in which the mother wakes up, knowing she is in labour. Instead of closing in and focusing on her contractions too early she takes a very long walk with her family. She then comes back and sits down to eat a meal, until she can't focus on eating any longer because her contractions are beginning to get stronger and longer.

The mother in the following case study used mindful hypnobirthing techniques through early contractions, but knew just the right time to go to hospital.

On 14 August, my waters broke at home about 3.45am, and I had some mild contractions for about 45 minutes. When making our way in the car to the hospital after 4.30am, my contractions went from five minutes to three minutes and increased in intensity. When I was examined at about 5.30am, to everyone's surprise I was 9 cm dilated and the baby was on its way! After a quick trip to the birthing suite, BJ was born about an hour and a half later at 7.45am. I used relaxation and visualisation tools between contractions, and used the time to rest and conserve energy. Later the midwives remarked that I was 'one chilled out mumma' during the delivery and were surprised at how far along I was when I got to the hospital as I was 'not behaving like other mothers-to-be in the transition period'. They also remarked that I had a high pain threshold. Looking back now, I realise that the Braxton Hicks or cramps I was having overnight in the days preceding my labour were actually pre-labour pains. I had used the relaxation techniques to deal with them and go back to sleep!

As your labour progresses you may find you turn your attention inwards more and more.

The image opposite may give you some idea of how your mind shifts from an externally focused state to an internally focused one. When contractions start, you may be able to cook some meals and do some washing or ironing, maybe even go for a walk or go shopping, just stopping to breathe through any contractions.

Then as they get longer and stronger or closer together you may find you want to stay in your home. This is often when women really nest, perhaps doing the last few things around the home to prepare. You might have a shower or a bath, and start to listen to

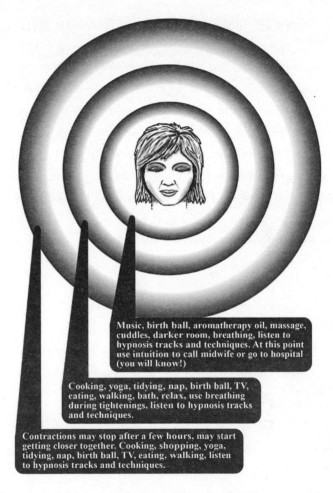

Music, birth ball, aromatherapy oil, massage, cuddles, darker room, breathing, listen to hypnosis tracks and techniques. At this point use intuition to call midwife or go to hospital (you will know!)

Cooking, yoga, tidying, nap, birth ball, TV, eating, walking, bath, relax, use breathing during tightenings, listen to hypnosis tracks and techniques.

Contractions may stop after a few hours, may start getting closer together. Cooking, shopping, yoga, tidying, nap, birth ball, TV, eating, walking, listen to hypnosis tracks and techniques.

As your contractions get stronger and longer, you will go more and more within yourself, perhaps unwilling to interact with those around you.

your hypnosis tracks. As the contractions get even closer together, you may feel as if they are waves and that you are just riding the waves, as you stay centred and focused in your birthing zone using breathing, affirmations and loving massage, and listening to your hypnosis tracks. When you reach your birthing zone, you should be in tune with the rhythm of your body, allowing your contractions to move through your body, bringing your baby to you.

MANAGING YOUR CONTRACTIONS

Each contraction may last from between 40 seconds to about one and a half minutes. Even if you are having three contractions every ten minutes, there will be around six minutes in every ten minutes for your body to rest. If you were in labour for ten hours contracting three minutes apart, your body would be contracting for three hours and resting for seven. When you are doing mindful hypnobirthing, the rest between contractions is important. If you are relaxed and floppy your muscles are able to let go between contractions rather than holding on to tension. Tension in your body between contractions can cause unnecessary pain.

Without tension, your body should relax completely between contractions, however intense those contractions are. A woman in labour who is relaxed between her contractions will have a very relaxed jaw and facial muscles. This is important because your jaw mirrors tension in the pelvic area. Relax your jaw and your pelvic area relaxes as well.

> **TIP:** Sometimes women can get very warm in labour. In a hospital it can be hard to get your hands on a tub of ice chips. Get four cheap flannels and soak them in water. Put each flannel in an individual food bag and freeze them. Before you go to the hospital take them out and put them in your hospital bag. They are really lovely on the back of your neck, your forehead or on your back during labour.

Putting your Practice to Use

By the time you go into labour and your contractions have begun, oxytocin will already have started to rise. Beta-endorphins will begin to flow, helping your body to relax into the rhythm of your contractions and helping you get into your birthing zone.

Contractions are like waves – you can feel one coming – so before a contraction you have a moment to collect and centre yourself, breathe deeply and focus. I often see women prepare for a contraction without realising, or even say, 'Here comes another one.'

As the contraction rises, you may feel tightness across your bump, and a strong squeezing. Sometimes in early labour your bump will simply harden, similar to a Braxton Hicks contraction. Just like a wave, your contraction builds up, peaks, then rolls away. Even if your contraction lasts for a minute and a half, it rises for only half of that, with just seconds at the peak. One woman said to me that when she felt her contraction rolling away, her body relaxed and the muscles in her legs had a deep sense of letting go. In her words, 'Like a gin and tonic goes to your legs at the end of a long day!'

Which Techniques Work Best During Contractions?

During contractions focus on your breathing, your mantra and your 'three, two, one, relax, relax, relax' (see page 46). If you need help to stay centred in your birthing zone use your hypnosis deepener (see page 48), perhaps asking your partner to count down for you. They can put a firm hand on your shoulder, which can be very reassuring and relaxing. At this point think of some of the anchors you have learned.

If you feel pressure or pain in your back, ask your partner to put pressure on your lower back just at the top of your buttocks. You can also use a massage roller ball in your lower back to apply pressure where you need it. If your partner isn't sure what to do, ask your midwife to help.

Warmth in the lower back can be very comforting. I always take a wheat bag with me; the hospital will warm it up for you. You can also put a couple of drops of your chosen aromatherapy oil on a warm wheat bag.

Movement, too, is helpful. You may find that you instinctively want to move during contractions, whether it's leaning over with your hips swaying from side to side, sitting on a ball rocking your pelvis, or even stamping from one foot to the other as I've seen some women do. Did you know that there are ancient belly dancing moves specifically for labour to help move baby down?

> **TIP:** Unpack baby's first outfit and put it in view. This can focus and relax you during contractions, reminding you of your baby on their way to you. Looking at something that reminds you that your baby is nearly here will also release oxytocin, the love hormone, helping with contractions and more feel-good beta-endorphins.

Should I Be Moving All the Time?

Movement is really important during labour as it helps baby move into a good position. The natural rocking movement of walking or swaying helps baby settle into the pelvis and wriggle down. Practising a walking meditation during labour is a great way for staying active and in your birthing zone. The following mindful walking meditation is a good exercise to use during labour, and to connect with the energy of contractions.

Walking Meditation

A walking meditation is a meditation that you practise while walking. It's a good mindfulness technique for labour as it enables you to stay in your birthing zone while moving around. As you are standing, become aware of your weight moving through the soles of your feet, connecting with the ground underfoot. Start walking, and with each step, be aware of the movement of your body as you walk, tuning into the rhythm of swaying gently as you walk. Bring your attention to the natural movement of your legs, your knees and your arms as you walk. Be aware of your breath as you walk, breathing in and breathing out. If you get a contraction while walking, pay attention to the energy rising within you; draw your deep breath from the ground, through the soles of your feet up through your body, allowing that energy to move through you. If something distracts you during your walking meditation, turn your attention back to the movement of your knees as they bend when you walk and the soles of your feet as they connect with the ground. You can also do this for 15 minutes a day during pregnancy.

There is nothing wrong with lying down for a bit if you feel tired or need a rest. If you lie on your left side with your headphones on listening to your hypnosis tracks, you can have a rest and your body will still have contractions. It's far better that you feel rested than weary and anxious about having to keep upright and moving.

Amy was in labour and had been having contractions every three minutes for around eight hours. She was at home and had done an active birth class, so knew the importance of movement. She walked around her kitchen, around her garden, around the fields nearby. Then, back in her kitchen, she turned and said to me, 'My feet hurt, I'm so tired.' I suggested she lie down for a bit, but she said she thought things would then slow down. I persuaded her that a rest would be a good idea, so we got her comfortable on her sofa, lying her on her left side with a cushion under her head and another between her legs. After a deep relaxation for over an hour she was rested, and an examination showed she had dilated a further 2 cm.

Connecting Mindfully with your Contractions

When you have a contraction, be in the moment. Think to yourself, 'Right now I am doing this, right now I can do this.' Remember that you only need to be able to be with one contraction at a time. If you can deal with one then you will be okay; don't worry about how many there will be, just focus on one contraction and on your breath. Turn your attention to that sensation rising and breathe into it, allowing it to move through you. Perhaps say to yourself, 'I can do this, I am doing it right now.'

Being in the present during labour is the perfect way to experience being in your birthing zone. When you are present, you are allowing the past to remain in the past and letting go of what may happen in the future. When you are focused on the present, you take each moment of labour, one breath or one contraction at a time.

Labour with Loving Kindness

Oxytocin is a love hormone; it responds to love, affection and familiarity. Birthing with loving kindness is certain to increase the levels of oxytocin and beta-endorphins. Being tender and affectionate with your partner between contractions can really help move things along and enables you to relax and let go. I've seen such tenderness between couples at births, and have very quietly stood back and allowed them to enjoy enveloping their birth and baby with love.

Remember, your baby was conceived through love, and the same hormone that made your baby will bring your baby into the world. Kissing, hugging and massage all help. You can ask for privacy if that's what you want, if it would help you to be more intimate.

> **TIP:** If labour is slowing down, or you wish to try and move things along for any reason, ask for some privacy from midwives and other people around. Have a massage and incorporate some breast massage and nipple stimulation into it. Midwives say that this really does the trick.

Birth Affirmations

You will have been listening to birth affirmations throughout your pregnancy. Putting those on now with your hypnosis tracks, either in the background or on headphones, will help keep you in your birthing zone. Your partner can also read them to you:

- Breathing slowly in and breathing slowly out.
- I trust and tune in to my body and to my baby.
- Breathing in I feel strong.
- Breathing out I let go.
- The more I relax the more my body softens and expands.
- The more my body softens and expands the more comfortable I am.
- I allow the energy of birth to move through me.
- I am centred and strong.
- Breathing in and breathing out.

- I take strength from those around me who I love and who are caring for me.
- I am filled with love for my baby.
- Each contraction wave is bringing my baby closer to me.
- My body relaxes between contractions and expands and opens during them.
- I am in tune with the rhythm of my body, with the rhythm of labour.
- I imagine the sensation as a comforting pressure nudging my baby down, down and down.
- My baby is surfing the waves, enjoying the gentle rhythm of labour.
- Breathing in and breathing out.
- As I breathe in I relax, as I breathe out I let go, relax, let go, relax, let go.

> **TIP:** Remember your headphones. In a busy environment they can really make a difference. As one mum said, 'I was amazed at how well it worked and how confident and calm I was throughout the labour. I found the best thing that worked was for me to listen to your hypnosis tracks on repeat with headphones in. When I was examined I took the headphones out and opened my eyes; the pain levels shot up and I couldn't wait to get the headphones back in my ears!

WHEN DO I CALL THE MIDWIFE?

If you are questioning if it's the right time to call the midwife, or others are saying, 'I think it's time we went in,' it's usually too soon. The right time will be when you say, 'I need to go now.' Once, when working as a doula, my client's husband said that they should go in. She replied, 'I don't really want to go yet.' Then two contractions later she said, 'Now, we need to go now. That one was different.'

It's very common for people to call the midwife or go to hospital too early. Studies show that it's often the partner's fear of responsibility, or the mother's own fear, that makes women go to the hospital too early or call the midwife too soon. While you may feel happier being in hospital, being there too early increases your risk of intervention.

One of my colleagues always says to the mother, 'If you can answer the door, offer to make me a cup of tea and biscuits, it's probably too early to call me.' A mother will be deeply within herself when she is in labour and her baby is nearly there, not thinking about making a cup of tea for visitors!

> **TIP:** If you have practised the techniques in this book you may not be responding in the way the health professionals expect. You may be much calmer and more relaxed than they would expect from someone who hasn't prepared mindfully. Make it clear that you are using hypnosis for birth, both when you ring up the unit and when you go in.

If you do want reassurance, you can go into hospital, have a check and then come home again, or call the midwife who can make a decision to stay or go. Studies show that for women planning a hospital birth an assessment before admittance can reduce the risk of intervention because the woman can go home reassured, and stay in the comfort of her home until the time is right to go back to hospital.

What if I'm Overdue?

There is a lot of pressure on women when they go over their dates, despite the fact that in reality only around 5 per cent of babies are born on their due date. Throw your due date out of the window and tell yourself that your baby will come when they are ready. Research shows that length of pregnancy can vary by up to five weeks and that older mothers are having longer pregnancies.

If you go over your due date, remember it's a guide, not the date your baby will be born on. You will not have reached what's known as 'term' until you reach 42 weeks. Just carry on as normal, and free yourself from any pressure to move things along. Remember that if you allow yourself to get stressed about it, you are increasing the levels of adrenaline that may prevent oxytocin rising and labour starting. Did you know that you have around a 95 per cent chance of going into labour before 42 weeks and around a 50 per cent chance of going into labour between 38 weeks and 41 weeks?

TIP: If you feel yourself getting anxious about going over your dates or feel under pressure to be induced, get some support and take time out to relax and let go. Reflexology, a pregnancy massage or acupuncture can be very helpful.

SUMMARY

- Trust your instincts.
- As labour starts, recognise it as a journey and relax or get on with other things between contractions in early labour.

- Take the opportunity to get final preparations done; get childcare in place if you need it; call your partner and let them know.
- Set up your room with the music and your anchors.
- Your partner can provide massage and loving cuddles that will help oxytocin flow.

14

MY BABY'S NEARLY HERE!

The power and intensity of your contractions cannot be stronger than you, because it is you.

Anon

You've called the midwife or arrived at hospital. Perhaps you know how far along you are. Remember, you can always choose to go home if you think you've gone in too early. Taking you through the basic steps of what happens when you call your midwife to your home or you go to hospital can help you prepare and become familiar with the process.

WHAT HAPPENS NOW?

If You Are Birthing at Home

A midwife will have a chat with you over the phone and ask questions about how far apart your contractions are and what's been happening. She'll more than likely pop along and take a look. She'll want to check on your baby, and do some basic observations on you such as taking your blood pressure and temperature. She may want to do an examination or she may choose just to observe you for a while. If she thinks you are in established labour she will stay and call another midwife. If she thinks you have a little way to go, or that you may benefit from a bit of space, she may leave, giving you her number to call if things change.

When You Arrive at Hospital

You'll arrive at the labour suite and be buzzed in. Most likely you will have rung ahead, so they will be expecting you. A midwife will meet you at the desk and take you either to a room or an assessment suite. An assessment suite might be a room with several beds like a ward or it might be quite a small clinical side room.

> **TIP:** Handing a copy of your birth preferences to the midwife who greets you is one of the first things you should do, even before assessment. It may change the way that they care for you from that first assessment and may make the assessment more in line with your birth preferences.

The purpose of assessment is to see how far along you are in labour and how you and your baby are responding. Usually at this point you will be offered an examination to check how far your cervix has dilated and the position of your baby. The midwife will also want to do basic observations like taking your temperature and your blood pressure. She may also assess you externally, observing how you are responding to contractions and how you are moving and breathing.

You have the option to turn down a vaginal examination at this point, but some studies show that in a hospital a clinical assessment on admission lowers the risk of intervention. This is because if they think you have a little way to go, they can suggest going home for a while. For some women it may be reassuring to have that check and then go home, especially if they are fairly close to the hospital.

When you are admitted to the unit, you will be given a room that you can make your own. Make yourself comfortable and ask for anything you need. Be confident in asking for what you want; part of the midwife's job is to support you in your wishes for the birth.

How You and your Baby Will Be Monitored

Throughout the book I've referred to undisturbed birth but if you are in a hospital for the birth, you may need to be familiar with more medicalised models of care during labour. How your labour is managed at this point will depend on several things: how well you and your baby are responding to birth; how far along you are when you are admitted; and the type of midwife you are assigned.

Both at hospital and home a partogram will be filled out to assess how your labour is progressing. A partogram measures, among other things, how you are dilating, time in labour, position of cervix, position of your baby, temperature, and how you are reacting to labour. Everything you decide or request will be put in your notes as well.

It's very useful to understand that an undisturbed birth is possible in a hospital. Even if your labour is higher risk and consultant led, you can still make choices that reduce intervention.

AN UNDISTURBED BIRTH

Undisturbed birth is exactly what it suggests – a birth when you are disturbed as little as possible. Disturbances can take the form of examinations and checks, chatter, background noise and lights. Taking steps to reduce these allows oxytocin, the birth hormone, to flow without interference from adrenaline. When you have an undisturbed birth you will birth your baby rather than having your baby delivered by someone else.

Mindful hypnobirthing is trusting that your body will birth in your own time. If all is well, do nothing. Keeping checks and examinations to an absolute minimum allows the space for your baby's birth to unfold in its own time and its own way, not according to charts based on averages. If you are at home you are more likely to fall automatically into a model of undisturbed birth.

Undisturbed Birth, in Hospital?

If you are in hospital you *can* have an undisturbed birth. You can still make choices that reduce interruption and disturbances – just make sure that they are on your birth preferences. I've been at plenty of births where the midwife has fully supported a mother having an undisturbed birth in a hospital. Usually she will say, 'Just press the buzzer if you need me, otherwise I'll pop in every 20 minutes to do observations on you and baby.' If she doesn't say this, tell her this is what you want.

Although the midwife will still chart progress on a partogram, she may start to navigate around the guidelines, adapting her practice to support the mother in how she is managing and responding to labour. She will intervene only if she thinks you or your baby may be compromised. There is no reason why your birth in hospital should not be treated the same way as a home birth. Make sure that you request a midwife who is happy to let things take their course and is interested in an undisturbed birth.

A MEDICALISED BIRTH

A medicalised birth is different from an undisturbed birth in that it is usually consultant led. However, some midwives may be more inclined to stick rigidly to more medicalised models of labour, particularly if a mother has not requested other approaches to her care. It can be the default approach to birth in many hospitals and birthing units.

A woman's progress is regularly checked against the partogram, and decisions of care are based on the picture that the partogram is giving rather than trusting the mother's ability to birth her baby in her own time and in her own way. It involves regular vaginal examinations, usually every four hours, depending on your hospital's guidelines. If labour slows down or isn't progressing as quickly as your midwife or doctor would like, you may be offered an amniotomy (having your waters broken) to help labour move along more quickly.

According to Dr Marsden Wagner, an American obstetrician:

The source of much of the confusion over normality found in medicalised birth is the mistaken idea that labour is something that happens to women rather than something women do. It is this idea which allows doctors to think they can intervene in what is happening rather than to assist the woman in what she is doing.

Even if you are higher risk and consultant led, you can take steps to ensure that your birth is as undisturbed as possible. Your midwife or doctor can still monitor you and your baby safely, making decisions to intervene only if there is a medical indication for it. When all is well you can allow the birth to continue, without needing to interfere in the pace and type of labour your body is dictating.

Interventions

I asked women which interventions they wished they'd known more about before giving birth the first time and have listed them below. These three very common interventions can make a difference to how you feel and to your state of mind during birth as well as your physical responses. Making yourself familiar with these, and reading up on the benefits and risks, can help you be more prepared and more in control of those choices.

Induction

If you go beyond your dates, you will be offered induction, usually at around 40 weeks plus 8 days, but maybe earlier if you are over 35 years old. Each hospital will have its own policy on induction so it's worth familiarising yourself with the one in your local hospital.

Sadly, induction is becoming more and more common in the UK. An audit of 17,000 births in Aberdeen showed that of the 32 per cent of women who had been induced, 28 per cent showed no reason for induction after the birth, raising concerns that women were unnecessarily being offered intervention. If labour is artificially started, it may mean that you are forcing your body to go into labour before you or your baby are ready.

There can be immense pressure placed on mums to induce labour before term at 42 weeks, even when there is no medical reason apparent. A client once booked me at 40 weeks as her doula because she didn't want to be induced. At 40 weeks and 7 days she started to get anxious and said, 'Women in our family can't birth spontaneously. My mother was induced with me, my sister with her two children and me with my first.' I said, 'If women in your family can't birth spontaneously you wouldn't be here. What about your grandmother?' She went on to have a fantastically quick birth at 42 weeks and 3 days.

Very often a woman will first be offered a pessary, a small tablet placed at the cervix. This releases prostaglandins that can stimulate labour. Sex is often recommended to start labour off, as sperm produces prostaglandins. If a pessary fails to get labour started, a woman may then be offered a drip containing artificial oxytocin.

If you are planning a birth with as little intervention as possible, it's important to understand that artificial oxytocin does not behave in the same way as your body's naturally produced oxytocin, and doesn't trigger the release of endorphins or your body's natural analgesia. Very often, labour induced by artificial oxytocin – or syntocinon as it's otherwise known – means that contractions may be more painful. Mothers who have had drip inductions sometimes end up in what's known as a cascade of intervention, meaning that one intervention may lead to another. For example, a drip induction can lead to pain relief choices, which may then lead to an epidural; and epidurals are linked to higher rates of instrumental births, which is when a doctor may use forceps or ventouse.

Having learned about the impact of adrenaline, think about how you may feel if you were told you were putting your baby at risk if you go overdue. It may create stress-releasing adrenaline and nor-adrenaline, potentially preventing the rise of oxytocin and the onset of labour.

If you are offered an induction, there are several sources of information that can provide you with independent advice. I would recommend the booklet produced by AIMS, the Association of Independent Midwives, called 'Induction – Do I Really Need It?', as well as familiarising yourself with the section on induction from the National Institute of Clinical Excellence (NICE) (www.nice. org.uk). This is the evidence-based guidance for those working in clinical practice. NICE writes the following about the choices being offered to women:

Healthcare professionals should explain the following points to women being offered induction of labour:

- *the reasons for induction being offered*
- *when, where and how induction could be carried out*
- *the arrangements for support and pain relief (recognising that women are likely to find induced labour more painful than spontaneous labour)*
- *the alternative options if the woman chooses not to have induction of labour*

- *the risks and benefits of induction of labour in specific circumstances and the proposed induction methods*
- *that induction may not be successful and what the woman's options would be.*

The guidelines also say that:

Healthcare professionals offering induction of labour should:

- *allow the woman time to discuss the information with her partner before coming to a decision*
- *encourage the woman to look at a variety of sources of information*
- *invite the woman to ask questions, and encourage her to think about her options*
- *support the woman in whatever decision she makes.*

There are many more stories of women today who, after reviewing the evidence, talked to their healthcare provider and decided to decline induction and, provided there were no medical indications for induction, to wait until their baby was ready to be born. You can discuss this option with your midwife.

Artificial Rupture of Membranes (ARM)

If your labour slows down, some interventions are offered such as breaking your waters, known as an amniotomy or artificial rupture of membranes (ARM). This is sometimes offered as a routine procedure in a medicalised labour to speed labour up and bring baby down further into the pelvis if they are 'too high'. As with anything, there are benefits and risks associated with this intervention. However, women are increasingly reporting that unnecessary rupture of membranes changes the course of their labour from one where they were managing well, to one that was much more painful. There are also a number of risks associated with an ARM, which, although small, can really alter the course of labour. A review of the available research states: 'the evidence showed no shortening of the length of first stage of labour and a possible increase in Caesarean section. Routine ARM is actually not recommended for normally progressing labours or in labours which have become prolonged'.

If labour has slowed down, consider the reason why this may have happened. If you are fine and the baby is fine, check your environment. Has something changed? Perhaps there has been a shift change and a new midwife; perhaps some different noises; perhaps for some reason you have been taken out of your 'birthing zone'. Consider the role of oxytocin and how easily it can be disturbed and slow labour down. Think about alternatives for getting labour moving again: adjust your environment so you feel secure and familiar; put your relaxation music on; use your hypnosis; perhaps try some aromatherapy or massage. If all is well, you can even go home. All these things offer a gentle and non-invasive alternative to ARM.

Remember, if you are well and baby is well, irrespective of whether they are 'high' or the bag is 'tough as old boots' as one mum was told, remember that your body is designed to birth your baby in its own unique way.

> Clare had a long labour with her first baby. She had an epidural, her waters were broken and she had forceps. When I arrived at the hospital for her second labour she was obviously in transition and her waters hadn't yet broken. When she was examined, the midwife said, 'You are 8 cm but your baby is still very high.'

Clare's response was, 'Yes, that happened in my first labour and they had to break my waters.' Her immediate thought was, 'Oh no, it's the same as last time.' I said to her, 'It's fine, you're doing well, your waters will break of their own accord, and your baby will come down.' Fifteen minutes later her waters broke and only 40 minutes later her baby was born.

Vaginal Examinations

Vaginal examinations can have a big impact on how a birth progresses and a mother's state of mind. They are often misunderstood. Most women I teach on my workshops have no idea that they have a choice when it comes to vaginal examinations (VE) – they assume that they have to have one and that knowing how far dilated you are is an indication of when your baby is going to be born. This isn't the case.

You may be surprised to learn that research shows VEs are just one aspect that assesses your progress. They need to be taken into consideration with several other factors. When you and your baby are responding well, then irrespective of how slow or how fast you are dilating, you are doing perfectly well.

Here are things that can help with making vaginal examinations a more positive experience:

- Having the same midwife undertake any examinations. Research shows that there is a considerable difference in measurements taken on the same woman by different people. Sometimes the difference can be as much as 2 cm.
- Make sure that you use your breathing and relax when you have an intervention. Put your headphones on, and don't feel the need to engage in conversation or small talk.

- Ask for minimal examinations. Studies show that you reduce your risk of intervention if you have an assessment at a unit before being admitted, but unless there is a medical indication there may be no need to make further checks.
- Choosing not to know how far dilated you are. For some women it can be deflating to find that they are 4 cm, and it's at that point they take pain relief. In fact, if you are 4 cm you may be 7 cm just a couple of hours later. Women dilate in very different ways.
- Trust that your body is taking labour at a pace that is comfortable and right for you. Stay in the present and in your birthing zone.
- Did you know that you can assess cervical dilation by the presence of a red/purple line that runs from your anus and extends between your buttocks? Research shows that this happens in a large percentage of women. This can give a good indication of dilation and how far down your baby's head is without an internal examination. You can ask your midwife about this as an alternative.

Good questions to ask if offered a vaginal examination are:

- Is there a medical need for me to have one?
- What difference could this make to my care?
- Why do I need to know how dilated I am now?
- Can it wait? Is there any other way I can find out?

WILL THE HYPNOSIS REALLY WORK?

Honestly? Yes, it will. I have used hypnosis in births that have been long and intense, with babies that are not in the optimum position. I've seen how powerful hypnosis is, and how being mindfully in each moment after great preparation can make even the longest labour an amazing experience. Second-time mums have said to me that the hypnosis I do with them during the birth is as effective as an epidural. I also know an anaesthetist who tells me that he only has to put a needle into the spine for the mum to say, 'Oh that feels amazing, I feel sooooo much better,' thinking the epidural has been administered. That's how strong your mind is!

Hypnosis is used in surgery all over the world and is an extremely effective form of anaesthesia. This extract describes Dr John Butler as he put himself into hypnosis for a hernia operation. You may feel a bit squeamish reading it, but it does show what your mind is capable of doing.

I told myself that, as the surgery progressed, I would feel more and more relaxed and my groin would feel numb to everything except touch and pressure. I repeated this to myself and felt myself drifting off.

But as I lay on the chilly, plastic-covered mattress of the operating table, my back began to twinge. I was worried the backache might distract me and was about to ask for a cushion when the surgeon made his first incision. This meant I wasn't fully in my hypnotised state, but even so I didn't feel a searing pain, just a minute amount of discomfort that soon disappeared as I re-established my own pain-killing thoughts. As the surgeon opened up my abdomen and stitched together my muscle wall to hold in my intestine, I let my thoughts drift, constantly repeating messages about numbness.

I could hear the surgeon speaking, but kept my eyes closed to focus on my own thoughts. I could feel his hands rummaging around inside me, which wasn't a pleasant feeling, but not painful. It was a legal obligation to have an anaesthetist in the room, in case of emergency, but all he did was monitor my vital signs, which stayed practically normal throughout.

Afterwards, I felt relieved that it was over – I hadn't felt the tiniest twinge of pain. I was offered painkillers, but it would have been strange to need them after what I had been through without them. Instead, I continued sending numbing thoughts to the area. I went home the same day, albeit walking gingerly to avoid tearing the stitches, and by the evening I was back at my desk.

What if I Need More Pain Relief?

If you are planning a hypnobirth, ideally you should have shifted away from the model of needing pain relief. One person said to me that if a woman can sit still enough to have an epidural in labour, she is certainly able to birth without the drugs; she just needs the right support.

Yet I also believe in a woman having the freedom to choose the option that is right for her, and to understand why she is making that choice. To be aware of all the risks and benefits is integral to having a positive and empowering experience. One thing I do know is how calm hypnosis makes a woman, even in the most challenging situations, and that one of the wonderful things about preparing psychologically is that you are prepared to make decisions and choices confidently and with a clear head, rather than acquiescing and handing over your choices.

There may be times when taking pharmacological pain relief may be more appropriate, and even then it is worth weighing up the risks and the benefits. For example, if you are really against a forceps delivery, then it's important to consider the impact of an epidural, which can increase your risk of an assisted delivery by 50 per cent.

If for any reason you feel you need other pain relief options, you can make them with an understanding of why you are doing it. Knowing the impact of certain interventions as well means you are fully aware of how they can affect a normal birth. I've listed both natural and pharmacological methods of pain relief below. Naturally, the use of non-pharmacological methods carries fewer risks as they are non-invasive.

Natural Pain Relief

TENS

TENS is a machine with a number of small pads fitted with electrodes that you can stick to your skin on your lower back. It feeds small electrical impulses into the nerve endings in that area, stimulating them. If you imagine your neural pathways are roads which can only carry one car at a time, the electrical impulses occupy those neural pathways, effectively blocking the road so the sensation of a contraction can't get through. You can buy them in some shops or even hire them.

TENS is based on the gateway pain theory. Although it's not clear exactly how it works, it is proven to have a strong placebo effect (meaning if you think it's turned on, even though it's not, you can have the same or similar effect as if it were on). I do know women who really benefit from it by using it as an anchor and focus. For some women, it helps them to shift focus away from the contractions. If you are using TENS make sure that you practise putting it on with your partner, as they can be quite fiddly. Make sure that your partner is familiar with how to use it when it's on. It can be quite helpful to get your partner to turn it up if you ask. Be aware that if you are choosing to have a water birth you won't be able to take the TENS machine in the pool with you.

Aromatherapy

Certain aromatherapy oils can be very effective at specific points during labour. Oils such as clary sage, lavender and mandarin are commonly used to help women relax during labour or speed labour up. When your muscles relax, pain reduces. You could visit an aromatherapist during pregnancy who will help you create an oil that is matched with your own feelings and expectations of birth. An aromatherapist will also give clear advice on what is safe to use and what isn't. In some hospitals aromatherapy is used by midwives; ask your midwife if this is offered in your local unit.

> **TIP:** Oils like peppermint are useful for nausea, both in pregnancy and during labour. Just put a few drops on a tissue and tuck it into your top or wave it under your nose.

Massage

Massage is really effective at reducing pain, helping you to feel connected and supported during labour. You partner can learn how to massage your legs, lower back and shoulders during labour.

> **TIP:** If you have the shakes or cramp in your legs, ask your partner to place their hands at the top of your thighs or your calves and, with long flowing strokes, run their hands down the entire length of your legs, right to the tips of your toes.

Acupressure and Reflexology

You can learn basic acupressure points and reflexology points. If this is something that interests you, make an appointment with a maternity reflexologist or an acupuncturist who can help you get familiar with important acupressure points to use during labour. Alternatively, there are many resources on line that will give you indications of pressure points in the body that are useful during contractions.

Water

Water is a popular form of natural pain relief during labour and is very compatible with mindful hypnobirthing. You can use a pool but a shower can be very comforting and is less likely to slow labour down. Getting in the pool may really work for some women but can slow labour down for others. If this happens to you, just get out, get warm and have a rest. Remember, if it does slow down, stay calm. It may take a little while for the oxytocin to rise again, but it will. You can take a bath early on as well, if you are at home and before you go into hospital. Whether you are in a pool or in a bath ask your partner to pour water over your bump or your back; this can be very soothing and relaxing. You can buy or hire pools to have in your own home if you are planning a home birth or just to enjoy using before you go to hospital; you may not want to get out and get in the car though!

Homeopathy

For some women homeopathy can be a useful way of managing emotions and sensations during labour. Many homeopaths offer a pregnancy and labour session, which includes loaning out a homeopathic birth kit.

Doula

A doula has bags of techniques and tricks up her sleeve to help with birth. Research shows that having a doula or continuous support reduces the need for pharmacological pain relief during labour.

Drugs Commonly Offered during Labour

Gas and Air

Gas and air is a mix of 50 per cent nitrous oxide and 50 per cent oxygen. It's breathed in through a small inhaler, is fast acting and disperses very quickly, within around 60 seconds. This is why during labour women are advised to take a breath as they become aware of a contraction rising and stop as it subsides. It's also called Entonox. There is very little research to show a negative impact of gas and air on your baby. However, if you watch a woman on gas and air, she tenses up her jaw, sometimes biting the mouthpiece. Tension in the jaw relates to tension in the pelvis, and a relaxed jaw means a relaxed pelvis. I've seen babies come much sooner in the final stages of labour when the gas and air is put to one side.

While gas and air can be very useful for some women, I've found others say that it distracted them too much and made them feel sick. Gas and air is available in a home or hospital setting.

Pethidine, Diamorphine and Meptid

You've spent nine months avoiding alcohol and certain foodstuffs, yet you are offered morphine during labour. Think very carefully about this. These are opioids and do cross the placenta, affecting your baby, although Meptid is thought to have fewer side-effects on baby. They are sometimes given to women who have a back-to-back baby or in very long early labours. Back to back is also known as occiput posterior and is when a baby's spine is facing to the back rather than the front. This means that there is increased pressure on the mother's back, which can cause pain and a longer early stage of labour. Dilation of the cervix may be slower as the baby's head will usually have to rotate to descend and press on the cervix to dilate it. Once baby has rotated though, labour can speed up considerably.

If a woman has had a very long early labour and needs to rest, pain relief such as pethidine can help her get the rest she needs for a vaginal delivery. However, a risk is that if your baby is born too soon after this is given it can cause respiratory problems and mean admittance to special care. Babies can be quite drowsy when the mother has had an opioid and it can affect breastfeeding. All of these drugs can cause vomiting in around one in three women and can make you feel spaced out. Some women say they feel very out of control and not able to speak or communicate what they want easily.

Epidural

An epidural is a local anaesthetic injected into the cerebrospinal fluid. It is a very effective painkiller, but can have a significant impact on the type of labour you may have. If you have an epidural you will be confined to the bed. A very low dose may, if you are lucky, allow some movement around the bed, but you will find it difficult to move off the bed.

It may slow down the second stage of labour as your muscles don't work as effectively to move your baby into the right position to descend. Coupled with lying down, this can reduce your pelvic outlet by up to 30 per cent, which is why epidurals result in a higher percentage of ventouse or forceps births. There are other side-effects such as losing bladder control and maybe needing a catheter. There are also more serious risks that are rare but do happen. For example, 1 in 100 women will get an epidural headache, which is a severe headache.

FINAL STAGES OF LABOUR

If you are in hospital, you will ideally have arrived at the perfect time and your baby will be born soon. In the final stages of labour you'll be deep in your birthing zone, allowing the contractions to move through you, focusing on your breathing. Your partner should already have prepared the room at the hospital or at home in the way you have planned with your anchors from Chapter 10. If you've arrived at hospital and things are moving along very quickly you won't have time to make a lot of changes in the room. If I arrive at hospital with a couple and the woman is well established in labour, I have my 1 2 3 room checklist:

1. Switch all the lights out.
2. Get the music on a dock, on headphones or in a CD player.
3. Drop a couple of drops of lavender oil on a tissue and tuck it into her top or put a couple of drops on the pillow.

As you move closer to birthing your baby, your contractions may get closer together; sometimes they may feel as if they are coming in waves on top of each other. You may even reach a point where your body may rest for up to 30 minutes, before beginning to move your baby down through the birth canal. This is sometimes referred to as the 'rest and be thankful stage'.

At this point in your labour your body's hormones naturally shift to increase levels of adrenaline and lower the levels of oxytocin. Adrenaline should be at very low levels during the earlier stages of labour; however, when your cervix is nearly fully dilated, usually from around 7–10 cm, you will have a natural surge of adrenaline. This stage is called 'transition'. This primal response makes a woman more alert and, if you were an animal in the wild, would be a sign that you need to find a safe place to birth as your baby will be here soon. Your baby also benefits from this final surge of adrenaline – their white blood count is increased, increasing their immunity; blood flow to the brain, heart and kidneys increases so that they are ready to function; and it also helps your baby's lungs prepare for that first breath.

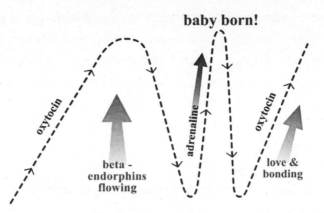

The undisturbed flow of oxytocin and adrenaline during labour.

When this happens, sometimes even hypnobirthing mums may want to run away. Some midwives report that it's not uncommon for mums to say, 'Right, that's it, I'm going home now,' or, 'I can't do this any more, give me the epidural.' I've also been with women and had absolutely no clue that they had entered that stage until they felt the urge to push or the head was being born.

I've heard some mums who misunderstand this phase of labour reflect angrily on the midwife and the experience of birth, saying that their request for an epidural was refused. In fact, rather than refusing it, the midwife recognised that it was too late to give an epidural. If this happens, remember in that moment that it's a sign your baby is nearly in your arms. One mother I knew said that when this happened, she recognised it and went within herself for an inner dialogue. Breathe, let go and know that you can do it, that you have done it; your baby is nearly here.

What if Labour Slows Down?

If labour slows down, firstly think about your environment. Has something changed? Are your anxiety levels rising? Do you have a new midwife? Is it suddenly noisier? Sometimes disturbances or changes can heighten your level of alert, reducing oxytocin and slowing down your contractions.

Stay calm if this happens. If you and your baby are well, there is no rush to do anything. Use the time to get some rest; perhaps lie on your left side on the bed, comfortable with your pillow and blanket and your partner nearby. Put your hypnosis tracks on and just drift off. You can also use your special place visualisation that you have practised with your partner (see page 83).

This is the story of a woman whose labour had slowed down but got it going again with the use of the techniques you are learning in this book.

On arrival at hospital I was hooked up to a monitor and brought a rather flat ball to use! It was really difficult to move around as I had before as every time I changed position the monitor fell off! After an hour and a quarter the midwife asked if she could examine me; I was still 6 cm and they discovered that the fore waters hadn't yet broken. The consultant wanted to break my fore waters and give me syntocinon to speed things up as they were concerned that the baby might swallow meconium. As the baby was fine at this point, I politely refused the interventions and my waters broke on their own five minutes later.

From about 4am until 7am I found that my breathing and lavender oil weren't quite enough so I had gas and air. At 7am, it appeared things weren't moving. Due to my moving around, the staff were struggling to keep a track of the baby's heart. It was suggested that I was examined and a monitor put on the baby's head. I agreed to the examination but again politely refused the monitor. My partner, Dave, and our doula said they would try to hold my monitor in place as I moved around. Unfortunately, the examination showed that things still hadn't progressed. I was starting to get tired and stressed at this point, so again I was offered syntocinon and we were given time to discuss things.

I was certain I didn't want the intervention so my doula suggested we ask if I could be taken off the monitor and move into the bathroom to try and regain some focus. I needed to take my mind off being in hospital, which is why I was struggling. Although the consultant was unhappy with this decision, our midwife was very supportive and spent a lot of time sitting on the bathroom floor listening to baby with a sonic aid!

During this time, Dave worked with me to talk me through the contractions with visualisations and breathing techniques we had learned from the hypnobirthing course. This really helped. However, after about three hours the consultants were very insistent that I needed to be constantly monitored as they couldn't fully assess the baby.

We moved on to the bed and Dave continued to talk me through my contractions. (The monitor still wouldn't stay in place!) About half an hour later my midwife asked if she could examine me again. I had reservations as I'd had quite a few since my waters had broken, but I also knew that we needed to know progress as I had been told that if things hadn't moved along by 1pm, I would have to have a section.

I was beginning to feel the need to push. When my midwife examined me she found that my cervix was fully dilated and the baby's head had started to move down. We then commenced pushing, during which I continued with my breathing and visualisations. Apparently, just before Molly was born I had begun to have enough, and as her head crowned I asked for ventouse to get her out! However, a couple of pushes later both her head and body shot out very fast.

BREATHE YOUR BABY INTO THE WORLD

You may have heard stories of women going red in the face from pushing or even seen it in films. It doesn't have to be like that. In fact, the prolonged chin on chest, deep breath, hold and push school of thinking is called the Valsalva Manoeuvre and is now known to increase the risk of complications in second stage. It can reduce oxygen levels, and increase carbon dioxide levels for both you and your baby. Studies show it makes no difference to the length of second stage. You won't need to be told to push; when you are ready your body will tell you to do it. Follow your body's lead.

> You can try this safely during pregnancy and even practise when you are on the loo. Clench your fist loosely and then put it to your lips. Blow out through your fist as if you are blowing up a balloon. Be aware of the way your breath is moving pressure in a downwards motion, but without tension in your body. This is a really great technique to use during second stage if you feel you need a bit more control and to exert a bit more pressure without straining.

Continue staying focused in your birthing zone. Even if you know you are 10 cm dilated, just continue to breathe and breathe and breathe, staying in the rhythm of your body. You may be aware of your baby moving down before the midwife is. I've lost count of the number of times mums have said to me that the midwife didn't think anything was happening and then suddenly the baby's head was there. As you breathe and relax, breathe and relax, your body will continue to bring your baby to you, in a natural peristaltic movement. Peristalsis is the same movement that your muscles in your intestines and bowel do as they move food through your body. It's like a pulsing wave that nudges your baby down and down, gently.

I just wanted to let you know that both Andrew and I firmly believe the hypnobirthing course was a huge factor in allowing me to stay calm and focused during Freya's birth. I did not even realise I was at the pushing phase until her head appeared – my body really must have taken over.

When you get the urge to push, go with it, but remember to take nice deep breaths in between.

MEETING YOUR BABY

The moment your baby slips into the world and on to your chest may be one of the most incredible of your life. You've done it! That little bundle of baby you are holding in your arms has been loved, nurtured and grown by you for the last nine months. You are connected with your baby in more ways than you can imagine. As your baby slips into the world, adrenaline drops and oxytocin starts to rise again, making sure that you and your baby are swimming in beta-endorphins and happiness. This helps establish bonding with your baby. If you are planning on breastfeeding you may be able to have your baby latching on within just a few minutes of birth, or it may take longer. Whatever happens, just enjoy the moment, stay calm and enjoy looking at and tuning in to your baby.

Take a Picture but Stand back from Facebook and Twitter!

These moments after birth are priceless. You will never get them back again. The feel of your baby's soft skin, meeting eyes with your baby, the feel of them curled up in your arms is something that should be locked in your memory. If you are not engaged in that experience mindfully you won't be able to easily recall it.

Your partner, your baby and you together are experiencing a unique and personal moment as your baby takes in you and the world outside the womb for the first time. By all means make sure you have a photo, but recently I've heard many midwives say that they want to ban phones from births. Those crucial bonding moments are lost as mothers are ignoring their baby and instead texting, sending Twitter updates, writing on their Facebook walls and sending photos to friends before the placenta has even arrived. Many babies now have a digital imprint before they have even left the hospital.

I know you'll want to share your news but allow yourself, your partner and your baby a quiet hour to really connect and bond with each other. Get to know your baby in that hour.

THE THIRD STAGE

The third stage is the part of labour when the placenta is delivered. In a birth that is undisturbed, you will have what is known as a physiological third stage. This means you allow your body to release the placenta rather than having an injection to speed up its delivery. Breastfeeding and skin-to-skin contact can help to release the placenta by triggering the release of oxytocin to contract the uterus. The cord stops pulsating, appears to lengthen and the natural release of oxytocin and prolactin triggers the uterus to contract and release the placenta.

It can take anything from minutes to over an hour for some women to birth the placenta naturally. Most take around 10 to 20 minutes. Some women choose to use their placenta afterwards to ingest as a smoothie or in capsules that are made for them, which is called 'placenta encapsulation'. This is because research shows that the hormonal concentrations in the placenta may help with milk supply, reduce post-partum depression and boost energy. Early studies in rats demonstrate that it contains pain relief properties. I have heard many women tell me that they have ingested the placenta and felt it really benefitted them, but admitted they would never tell their friends! In some cultures, such as in Malaysia, they bury the placenta, giving the tissue that is genetically identical to the baby the burial it rightly deserves.

In a medicalised third stage you will be given an injection that helps the uterus contract and release the placenta. The cord will be cut almost immediately, although research shows this practice is now slowly changing in many units in the UK to allow for delayed cord clamping. This allows baby to receive more of their blood from the placenta and is proven to have health benefits for baby. You can still request for the cord to be left until it has stopped pulsating, even if you have a managed third stage or if your baby is born early or, in some cases, by Caesarean. You may be recommended a managed third stage if you have had any complications during pregnancy or labour.

SUMMARY

- Allow labour to follow its own path and trust in that journey.
- Use your techniques to manage your contractions and rest between them.
- Stay in the present. 'Right now you can do it, in this moment all is well.'
- Create a loving and tender environment to welcome your baby.
- Have skin-to-skin contact and enjoy getting to know your baby.

15

WHEN THINGS TAKE A DIFFERENT PATH

In this chapter I'll cover some of the unexpected choices and complications that women may be faced with during labour. These will give you a flavour of how mindful hypnobirthing techniques can be applied to any situation, how choices are made and how couples navigate their birth journey. All women are different, and birth can throw a curve ball, which may mean you rethinking your preferences and presenting you with choices at a fork in the road. This may be anything from the position of baby through to a Caesarean birth.

When you have to make an unexpected choice because of the route your birth has taken, you won't always remember the circumstances and reasons why you made that choice. Hindsight can create a very different picture and our memories are unreliable, especially when you are making decisions from a place of emotion and maybe fear.

First of all take a deep breath and refer to your BRAINS questions (see page 96). If it happens during your pregnancy, you have time to do some research. Even in the early stages of labour your partner can do some research online that can help guide your questioning.

When you make a choice, one that you think you may question later, make sure that you have time to go through these three points.

Even write them down if time permits. It will remind you that you did the best you could based on the information you had:

1. These are the facts I was given.
2. This is the choice I made.
3. These are the reasons I made that choice.

The following examples of common complications illustrate that there are alternatives to many of the choices that arise. They also show how the hypnosis techniques you have learned in this book will stand you in good stead, whatever happens.

LOW-LYING PLACENTA

Many women don't think there is much point in practising for a hypnobirth if they are told at the 20-week scan that they may have to have a Caesarean birth because their placenta is low-lying. However, if your placenta is not covering the neck of the womb it is unlikely to be a problem. Imagine that your uterus is a deflated balloon; stick a small piece of Blu Tack near, but not over, the neck of the balloon. Now blow it up. You'll see that as the balloon gets bigger, the piece of Blu Tack moves further and further away from the neck of the balloon. The same is true of how your uterus grows. It's actually very rare to have what is known as placenta praevia at term. Around 98 per cent of women who are told that they have a low-lying placenta at their 20-week scan will be completely normal at term.

The hypnosis techniques you learn will benefit you and your baby even if you do have to have a Caesarean birth (see page 203), so it's well worth learning the techniques if you are told you have a low-lying placenta.

BABY'S POSITION: BREECH AND POSTERIOR

Getting your baby into a great position for birth will help the cervix dilate more quickly and baby move down. Sometimes babies are in more awkward positions, maybe breech (head up) or back to back (baby's back is facing backwards rather than towards the front). You can help prevent this by making sure that you sit well during pregnancy; avoid slouching on a sofa and find positions in which your back is straight and you are leaning forward slightly. Birth balls can be great for sitting at a desk.

> **TIP:** Kneeling chairs can be a good option during pregnancy when sitting at your desk, reading or watching television. The chair will straighten your spine and tip your pelvis forward, and is particularly good in later stages of pregnancy by taking pressure off your back. Less pressure is placed on the womb as the angle between the trunk and thighs is increased. It is great for relieving backache and actually helps to strengthen the back in preparation for birth.

If your baby is breech, you do have the option of a vaginal birth, depending on the type of breech. More and more units are supporting breech births. Remember, if your baby is breech they can turn even at the last minute. The best thing you can do is relax, listen to your hypnosis tracks and trust that baby will do what is best for them.

During labour, active movement can help baby move into a good position, especially if baby's back is aligned with your back. Lying down on a bed will make it harder for baby to swizzle into the best position for birth, so movement such as rocking or bouncing on a birthing ball is a better option.

You may find that a visit to a chiropractor or an osteopath that specialises in birth can be really helpful before labour, just to correct any misalignments.

PREMATURE RUPTURE OF MEMBRANES (PROM)

In around 8–12 per cent of full-term pregnancies, from 37 weeks, a woman's waters will break before labour starts. This is known as premature rupture of membranes (PROM). Around 95 per cent of women will go into labour spontaneously within 24 hours. Most hospitals have a policy to induce someone after 24 hours to reduce the risk of infection. Remember this is a policy, not something you have to do. You have to weigh up the true risk of infection with the risks associated with an induction, especially if you are intending to have an undisturbed birth. Research shows the difference in neo-natal infection between induction and expectant management increases very slightly from 0.5 to 1 per cent. Expectant management is to wait but to make basic observations.

If you choose not to be induced you will:

- be informed of the risk of infection
- be advised that delivery should take place in a hospital
- be advised to stay in for observation for 12 hours after the birth

Expectant Management

If you choose to wait you will be advised to:

- check your temperature every four hours and let your midwife or the hospital know if your temperature is over 37.4, if you are feeling unwell, or if there is any change in the colour or smell of your waters

- have a foetal heart rate and foetal movement assessment by a midwife every 24 hours
- meet a senior obstetrician for further discussion if you are not in labour after 72 hours

An induction can be arranged by your midwife if you request it.

RAISED BLOOD PRESSURE

Your blood pressure will be measured on a regular basis during your pregnancy. Increased blood pressure can be connected to complications such as pre-eclampsia, which is why it's regularly checked. A midwife will be concerned only if it goes above 140/60 or is accompanied by other symptoms.

The biggest problem for women is something called White Coat Syndrome. This is when your heart starts racing when you have tests done at a doctor's and is because of anxiety. Research shows that women are more likely to suffer from White Coat Syndrome in pregnancy, and that as many as 32 per cent of pregnant women may be affected. If you have high blood pressure in the absence of any other symptoms, use your hypnosis techniques to relax and calm yourself when you have your blood pressure taken.

Ella started her labour at home and was planning to go into the midwife-led unit when she was ready. The midwife came to her home to do the checks, but found her blood pressure high; the midwife moved her to a lying-down position and took it again. It was still high. I suggested to Ella that we did a deep relaxation and her blood pressure went down to normal. We repeated this later, preventing a transfer to hospital.

Sometimes a doctor may suggest an induction if your blood pressure rises at term. One woman I know didn't want to do this and asked, 'Is there an alternative?' The doctor replied, 'Yes,' and gave her some tablets to bring it down. She went into spontaneous labour 10 days later. You can request for the community midwife to take your blood pressure in your own home if you think that this would make a difference.

GOING OVER YOUR DATES

Going over your dates is one of the most common reasons for an intervention, in the form of an induction. I've discussed this in more depth on page 173. Babies come in their own time; if all is well your baby might need a little longer. Your body will trigger labour when you are both ready. Before agreeing to an induction, do lots of research and really weigh up the risks associated with induction versus waiting.

If you want an undisturbed birth you should consider the implications of an induction to your care and to the birth. You can have a normal vaginal birth without medication with an induction, but it can be more painful than when you go into labour naturally, and the risks of falling into a cascade of intervention are higher.

Here is a visualisation if you are overdue.

Imagine an apple tree, rich with fruit. There is one particular apple you need to get down; it looks red and juicy and ripe. You really want that apple and you want it now. You've waited through winter, seen the blossom in the spring and now it's autumn and that apple is so big and round. It looks ready. You get impatient; every day you come out to the tree to see if the apple has fallen but it hasn't. Eventually, one day you decide enough is enough; if that apple doesn't fall today then there must be something wrong with it. If it stays up there much longer it won't be as red and round and juicy. You have to give it a helping hand.

So the next day you shake the tree trunk with all your might, but the apple doesn't budge. In the end you think, 'Maybe if I climbed the tree I would get it sooner.' The tree is high, and you realise that if you were to climb the tree you would be tired, it would be hard work, your legs might get scratched and there is no guarantee you would reach it safely or the apple would be easy to pick once there.

So you sit under the tree to contemplate and reflect on your apple. You see the beauty of that apple, so perfect in its surroundings. You become still and patient under the tree, aware of the peace and quiet in this beautiful place, knowing deep down that the apple will fall from the tree when it is ready.

Then one day while you are quietly clearing the leaves from the grass around the tree the apple falls, right in front of your feet on a soft clump of moss. You bend down and lift it up; it's perfect without a blemish. You bite into that apple and are amazed at how perfectly sweet it is, that by leaving that apple to fall from the tree when it was time you let it ripen just as it was meant to.

This is a story of a client of mine.

Amanda hired me as a doula at 40 weeks. She had started to feel anxious and had come to see me for hypnosis to try and get things moving. Her first birth had been a very long induction at

41 weeks and 4 days. She didn't believe she could go into labour naturally but she decided to let things take their course; her baby would come when he was ready, and hiring me as her doula would keep her focused.

Sure enough, Amanda went over her dates by a week and had a meeting with the consultant. She said she'd rather not be induced if all was well but to wait. All was well, and when she reached 42 weeks she began going into the hospital for regular monitoring. At 42 weeks and a day she was asked to pop in and see the consultant on her way out after the scan. I received a distraught phone call from her, saying she was having a 12 lb baby. The consultant wanted to give her a Caesarean on the spot but Amanda agreed to go in for an induction in two days.

The night before her induction I got a call at 4am. A drowsy Amanda said, 'Don't rush, there's plenty of time,' as I dashed out of the house. After a very quick labour, her little boy was born at 7.30am weighing 9 lb 10 oz.

PRE-TERM LABOUR

If you go into labour before 37 weeks it's classed as pre-term. If your waters break before 37 weeks, you won't be induced but the hospital will use expectant management (see 197) and you may be expected to stay in hospital. You will be monitored very carefully and may be given steroid injections to help mature your baby's lungs. No one fully understands why some babies are born early, but even if this happens to you the hypnosis techniques you have learned can help immensely. Not only will they keep you calm, they will also benefit your baby.

You can use the hypnosis tracks to get some rest and relaxation if you are on a ward. You can also help by getting the room how you want it during the birth.

> My due date was estimated as 22 June. However, our baby had other plans and at 36 weeks my waters broke. I had originally been booked into the birthing centre and had my heart set on a water birth. When I got to the hospital I was told that because I was early there was no chance of going to the birthing centre. To further add to my disappointment I was told I would have to be admitted to a ward straight away, which scuppered my plans to stay at home as long as possible.
>
> I had to stay on the ward and, 36 hours later, my labour started naturally in the early hours of the morning. Even though it was not how I'd envisaged my labour to be, I used all of the techniques you taught throughout the course to keep a positive mindset and remain relaxed and focused. It was difficult as I was on a ward with three other women all in various stages of labour. However, I used your advice and listened to the CD, closed my eyes and used the breathing techniques when the contractions arrived. I took my birth ball, yoga mat, pillow and green fig oil spray – these all really helped to make me feel relaxed and in control throughout the first part of my labour. I stayed off the bed (my partner Alex made sure of that by lying on it while watching television!)
>
> I listened to my body and when the contractions became very intense I asked to be checked. I was 5 cm dilated and was taken down to the delivery suite. Alex set up the room for me to make it feel comfortable and it really helped. I felt so relaxed and this gave me the confidence to feel I could deliver my baby with minimal intervention.

I used gas and air and my breathing techniques, and three hours later our son was born. When he came out he was really calm. I sat with him on my chest and had a natural third stage; my placenta came out 20 minutes later. I can honestly say that I think without all the techniques we learned from your course and from my antenatal yoga classes, my labour would have been a lot different. Alex took on board all the advice from the course and as a result was an amazing birth partner.

CAESAREAN BIRTH

If you have a planned or unplanned Caesarean birth you can use hypnosis techniques to help you stay centred and focused. Many mums I know have had very positive experiences, knowing that by preparing well for their birth they did the best they could for themselves and their baby. When you prepare well, and make the right choices for you, you will more than likely reflect on the birth with pragmatism rather than regret.

Hypnosis for birth is not just about undisturbed vaginal birth; it gives you the tools to have a positive experience, whatever birth you have. This will help you bond and connect with your baby well, however your birth went. The practice you do also benefits your baby; taking time out to relax and release stress, and to prepare for parenthood emotionally, will make a difference to you in the early days after the birth and in the long run.

In a Caesarean birth the hypnosis techniques can help while you are having your epidural or spinal, the injection that numbs you from the waist down. Use your breathing techniques to centre yourself and to stay calm. Depending on your own circumstances, you can ask to have your baby skin to skin and delayed cord clamping. You can also request for the drapes to be lowered so you can learn the sex of your baby, if you don't already know.

Once in surgery I was actually very relaxed. My partner Matt and I chatted to the anaesthetists and were really excited to meet our baby soon. I think Matt and I held our breath with him until we heard his first cry. He was then handed straight to Matt who held him by my head for the rest of the operation. I barely noticed what the doctors were doing as we gazed at our gorgeous new son and the midwife took some pictures of the three of us. I'd had more than 40 hours of labour followed by the Caesarean section, but I still didn't feel at all tired – I was on top of the world to have our little boy with us!

It may not have been the ending to the birth that we had hoped for, but it was really special nonetheless. I can honestly say I enjoyed labour and am happy that when things didn't go the way I hoped I remained in control and chose the intervention that I was happy with. I was amazed at how well the hypnosis techniques worked during labour and not once did I even consider needing any drugs to help me – it all felt totally manageable and an amazingly empowering experience.

SUMMARY

- Whatever path your birth takes, the mindful hypnobirthing techniques you have learned will benefit you and your baby.
- Remember that even if things change you still have choices.
- Take time to reflect on what they might be, and do research if you need to.

PART 3

WELCOMING YOUR BABY TO THE FAMILY

16

WELCOME HOME

Birth is the beginning – the beginning of life, the beginning of parenthood, the beginning of family.

Kathy McGrath

If you have had a hospital birth, depending on your birth and the hospital you can leave anything from hours to days after your baby has been born. When your labour has been quick and free of intervention you can choose to be discharged within hours. If you have had a surgical birth or intervention you may need to stay in from one to three nights.

If you are at home, the midwife will leave when she has cleared up and is happy that all the checks on you and your baby are fine. Then you can snuggle up in bed and enjoy your baby.

THE FOURTH STAGE

Those early days and weeks after your baby has been born can be called the fourth stage, or 'babymoon'. This is a time to slow down, accepting the slower pace of life and getting used to life as a newly expanded family. Get ready for the fourth stage before baby is born; this can set you in really good stead and means that you will glide seamlessly from the birth into those early days without feeling that you are always catching up on yourself.

Even though they may have prepared really well for the birth, new parents often aren't prepared for these early days. I've yet to meet a new parent who isn't tired and who realises that it takes a lot longer to do things than it did before their baby was born. This time will pass, and baby will settle into a routine of their own accord, but slowing down and limiting what you do can make it much easier. You can use this time to mindfully connect with your baby and really get to know them without distraction.

For baby, too, it's an important time when they are learning to adapt to a completely different environment; too much activity can overstimulate your baby. Think about how sensitive they are to noise after being in the womb with softened sounds and vibrations. Imagine how it must be for your baby being handled by unfamiliar people all the time. Babies don't even know what people are at this stage; they are just huge lumbering shadows moving about.

If baby is unsettled, try putting on the hypnosis tracks. Your baby associates them with feeling relaxed. When you listen to them in pregnancy those relaxing hormones crossed the placenta, so your baby will be conditioned to respond to them. One parent I know has been through two CDs with her children.

Your Hormones Settling Down

In those early days your hormones will be shifting and settling down. It's not uncommon to get a bit teary, but if you feel as if you aren't coping or are struggling get in touch with your health visitor or your GP. There is help and support for mums.

If you have prepared emotionally you may have a smoother transition into parenthood. It can help to talk through your emotions, addressing them in pregnancy. It is also valuable to have a solid support system so you don't expect too much of yourself, to be flexible, and most of all to take time out for yourself every day.

Stress-free Breastfeeding

If you have chosen to breastfeed you'll need space to connect with your baby and tune in to their cues for feeding. The more relaxed you are the easier your milk will flow. The same hormones that affect birth affect breastfeeding, so when you are comfortable, relaxed and feel private your body will release oxytocin and prolactin, triggering milk flow. If you are stressed about feeding or feel you are being watched, you trigger adrenaline, which slows your milk flow. You can use the techniques you used during your birth to help you relax when you are feeding. If you need help ask your midwife or health visitor. There are many other groups who can offer support, such as La Leche League and the National Childbirth Trust, as well as private lactation consultants who run breastfeeding groups. You can find their details in the Resources section (see page 232).

KEEPING CENTRED IN THOSE EARLY WEEKS

There are a few things you can do to help yourself prepare for the fourth stage. Remember, you are not being selfish if you choose to decline visitors; you are putting your family first. You are not being lazy if you are not dressed before midday; you are slowing down the pace and giving your attention to your baby. Do what is best for you and your baby. When you feel you are ready, you can start reaching out to local postnatal groups and perhaps meeting up with other mums you met on your antenatal classes.

Here are some tips to help you in the early days and weeks:

- Prepare meals in advance and put them in the freezer.
- Set up a standard essentials list on an online shop so you can shop in seconds.
- Accept help, whether it's cleaning or cooking or taking baby for a walk so you can get some rest.
- Leave housework and choose sleep when you have some free time.
- Limit visitors to a specific time. People can work around you, not you around them. Think about a 'do not disturb' sign for your front door; you'd be amazed how many people just 'drop by'.
- Get a sling so you can get on with things while your baby is soothed by being close to you.
- Before your baby is born take a class on preparing for these early days (see babycalming.com).

Remember, when you are calm your baby will be soothed. Your baby will mirror you and be watching you all the time. The techniques you have learned for the birth will also help in the early days. The 'three, two, one, relax, relax, relax' exercise (see page 46) and your breathing exercises will also help centre you.

On the opposite page a brief mindful Mamma exercise that will help you calm and connect with your baby. You can copy this and put it somewhere you can see it regularly.

Soothe

Smile and speak kindly to yourself and to your baby.

Observe your own feelings and emotions.

Observe your breath, slow down your breathing.

Tune in to your baby, tune in to your instincts.

Hold your baby, mirror your baby.

Exhale any stress, and as you breathe in envelop your baby with love.

SUMMARY

- Your baby is here! Enjoy your baby. Allow your new family the space to connect quietly and get used to each other.
- Learn to recognise your baby's cues without too many external distractions.
- Leave the dishes in the sink and answer your baby's cry.
- Get help if you need it but use these early days to adapt.
- Your pace of life may be a lot slower; allow yourself time to get used to it.

BIRTH STORIES

SOPHIE'S BIRTH: A HOME WATER BIRTH

Sophie Faith Banks was born in water at home on Monday 4 February 2013 at 5.50pm, weighing 8 lb 7 oz. This is the story of her amazing birth.

I woke at around 3am on Monday 4 February and felt wet. I went to the bathroom and I believed my waters had gone. I tried to go back to sleep but was getting contractions on and off and wasn't comfy in bed, so I got up and came downstairs and watched telly while sitting on my birth ball. By about 6.30am I felt that the contractions were getting a bit closer so I woke Dave up and asked him to start timing them. They were about 20 minutes apart.

We pottered around with Molly and had some breakfast and I spent most of my time on the ball as it was the most comfortable place to be. We rang Stephanie (our doula) and she arrived about 10am, by which point I was baking cakes with Molly as she was getting bored as we'd decided to keep her off nursery. I was still contracting regularly and using the breathing techniques I'd learned at the Mindful Mamma class to relax through them.

By about midday my contractions were coming every three minutes and I was seated on a chair with Stephanie massaging my back. As the contractions were getting closer and longer, Dave started to get the birth pool ready with Molly before taking her over to her friend's house while Stephanie and I had some lunch. Things slowed down a little while I ate but went back to every three minutes afterwards, so we decided to call the midwife at about 2pm.

The midwife arrived just after 3pm. I was in the dining room breathing through my contractions while Stephanie continued to massage my back. Everything was going well and I was well into my birthing zone. The midwife spoke to Dave and wanted to examine me, so reluctantly I came out of my zone and went into the living room – by this point it was 3.45pm.

I was a little disheartened as, despite my birth preferences clearly stating that I didn't want to be told of my progress, she informed me I was 4 cm dilated while she was still examining me and that my waters hadn't actually gone. Her shift was about to end but she asked me to provide a urine sample before she left. Dave and I went up to the bathroom and we spent about half an hour up there so that I could re-establish my breathing and get back into my zone – I didn't even try to provide a sample! During this time the new shift of midwives arrived.

After our time in the bathroom I could feel pressure building and said that I felt the baby wouldn't be long. I came back to the dining room and Dave spoke to the midwives who were very happy to leave me to get on with things. I wasn't really aware of time but I'm told that I only got into the pool at about 5.20pm as both Stephanie and Dave felt I was in transition.

I remember being totally relaxed in the pool, breathing through the contractions and visualising my baby moving down. Dave was sitting at the side of the pool talking to me, and Stephanie asked if I could feel baby's head. I could but she was still a few centimetres inside. The midwives came in and checked the pool and Stephanie went to get some more hot water as they said it was too cold.

While Stephanie was in the kitchen I looked down and Sophie was floating in the water in front of me! I had obviously breathed her out and she had taken everyone by surprise. I wish we had a video so we could see what had happened but she must have swum up to me. I lifted her out of the water and was passed my glasses so that Dave and I could see her sex for ourselves. She was a perfectly healthy little girl, covered in vernix. There had been no shouting, no pushing and no drugs.

I left the pool for the third stage and after about half an hour of being fed cake and tea, my placenta was delivered naturally, still attached to Sophie. Just over an hour after Sophie's birth I had a lovely bath. Molly came home briefly to meet her new sister before going back to her friend's for a sleepover. By 9pm, Dave, Sophie and I were tucked up on the sofa eating egg and chips.

SAMSON JACK: A HOSPITAL BIRTH

Samson was born at a hospital further away than Jo would have liked. Despite this, she and her partner stayed calm throughout the journey and when they arrived Samson was born in just a few pushes.

Our baby was due on 6 March 2012. This never seemed like the right date to us and we felt that the baby would arrive on 10 March from the beginning. I wanted a drug-free birth and a lot of my friends had used hypnobirthing to varying degrees of success. I have been frightened of drugs and medicines ever since I had my drink spiked at 19; I am frightened of the effect it may have on my body and fearful of being out of control. I wanted very much to be in control during labour, to remember every second of bringing my baby into the world and not to be afraid.

I have used mindfulness meditation in my everyday life for over 10 years now and was very excited to find a course using the techniques for labour. My other half was quite sceptical though, and not at all convinced that the power of the mind could overcome extreme pain. We found the course itself brilliant: the videos, practice and simplicity of the meditation won over my other half and we left keen to put the scripts and techniques into practice. We wrote a script together and the other half recorded it on to my iPhone so I could practise when he wasn't around. I used the music and script almost every day from seven months pregnant and multiple times a day in the three weeks leading up to my due date.

Predictably, 6 March came and went without a baby and I began to feel twinges on the evening of 9 March. I sat for the whole evening on my birthing ball and meditated to relax, sending the other half to bed early, just in case. By midnight I was feeling nothing so decided to go to bed. At 2am I woke up feeling some sort of pain, but it wasn't intense, so I wandered downstairs, put on a film and sat on the ball. Fairly quickly I realised I was having regular contractions, but it wasn't that painful. We'd decided to delay using any mindfulness techniques until the pain ramped up.

By 4am I was quite uncomfortable and woke up the other half. We phoned the hospital to book in (normal practice in Brighton) and I got into bed. By now I was having quite strong, short contractions but feeling nothing in between. We used 'three, two, one, relax, relax, relax' to relax my body and we both fell asleep between contractions, even if only for a few minutes. We both felt very calm and prepared; we were excited about meeting our baby and knew it was time for the baby to arrive. By 9am it was too uncomfortable to lie down any more, so we got up and I used the sofa to lie on between contractions and to lean on during them. By now, I had a lot of pressure in my upper legs, so stroking turned into hard rubbing which really helped to relieve the pressure.

Around 10am I stood up for a contraction and my waters went all over the living room floor. This really did take us both by surprise and there was a moment of panic. We calmed down using 'three, two, one, relax, relax, relax' and phoned the hospital. It was then we discovered that Brighton Hospital was closed for any new admissions and we'd need to go to Haywards Heath, a 30-minute journey from our house (Brighton Hospital is around five minutes away). The midwife said we should leave right away to be assessed. I felt fine and would happily have got into the bath, but the other half wanted to leave straight away so we packed up our things and got into the car. We put on the music that I had been using to relax. I felt calm and in control and knew this was the final journey we needed to make to meet our baby. The music was exactly the right length to take us from our house to the hospital.

Less than five minutes after getting into the car I had a new sensation and, after a second, realised I was getting the urge to push. I asked my other half if we were nearly there as I needed to push; he went pure white and said, 'Hold on.' He calmly drove to Haywards Heath, although afterwards admitted he didn't really know the way and we took a few detours.

We arrived at the hospital at midday, abandoned the car at A&E as we'd been told and found the delivery suite. We met our lovely midwife, Dionne, and she asked to examine me. Immediately she said she could see the baby's head and that I was 10 cm dilated and about to give birth. We were both quite shocked, but also relieved that that the baby was about to arrive. We didn't have time to move the car; the baby wasn't going to wait!

I tried various positions to push. The talking of the midwives was quite distracting and my contractions slowed down. I ended up standing up. My partner was fully involved, telling the midwives to let me get on with it and holding on to me to keep me standing. Four pushes later, at 1pm, our beautiful baby arrived, screaming, into the world. It was a wonderful sound. My partner told me we had a boy and cut the cord. I can still remember the sound of his voice as he told me we had a son, full of pride and cracking with emotion. I was handed our son and he sat in my arms, quiet now and looking round at the world. He was just perfect.

We didn't have a chance to use everything we planned, such as the lighting and music, and our birth plan never even made it out of the car! But I think the techniques were so successful for us that labour progressed more quickly than we'd ever imagined and was manageable.

It was the birth we had hoped for: both of us doing it together, supporting each other, without any fear or intervention. We named our son Samson Jack and he arrived on 10 March as we'd been predicting from the beginning. He remains a happy, calm little boy and is now almost 10 months old. I also think that our calm birth helped us so much in the early days, particularly with feeding. I breastfed Sam from the beginning without any problems and strongly believe that being calm and believing my body could do it helped us both get the hang of it.

I can't thank you enough for the techniques you have given us. We wouldn't hesitate to use them again should we have more children and have recommended you to our friends. The birth of our son is a day we remember every second of and will cherish forever. Thank you.

MAYA'S BIRTH

Cat's pregnancy wasn't straightforward, but Cat used the hypnobirthing and mindfulness techniques really well and went on to have a home birth.

This is the story of the birth of my beautiful daughter. After much research my plan was to have a doula and a home water birth in a calm and relaxed atmosphere. My husband was dubious at first and questioned why we needed a doula, but after talking to Sophie he understood that she was there for both of us.

We also took the Mindful Mamma hypnobirthing course as we were both keen to learn how to have a relaxed and calm birth. The course was a full day and opened our eyes to how birth can be an enjoyable experience. We left the course feeling positive and excited about our up and coming birth.

A few months into my pregnancy I was referred to the consultant as my BMI was just slightly over the cut-off point. He said that I would need to have a diabetes test done and also have regular scans in case my baby was large.

At 28 weeks I went for my diabetes test. When my tests came back I was told that I was on the borderline of gestational diabetes and would need to take my blood five times a day and watch my diet. After taking my bloods for over two weeks I had all normal readings. I discovered that the hospital I was at had a very low cut-off point for gestational diabetes, and if I had been at several other hospitals within my area it wouldn't have been an issue. This was crazy because the hospital wanted to induce me at 38 weeks because of the risk of a large baby. This was despite the fact that babies in my family, and in my husband's, have always been small. My previous scans, too, had indicated a small baby. My husband is Indian and Indian babies are on average 300 g smaller than European babies, but the hospital wasn't willing to take this into account as they couldn't guarantee that he was the father.

The hospital advised that I would need regular scans so I agreed to have one extra scan. After this, everything changed as they were now worried that my baby was measuring small, which they feared was due to a problem with the placenta or cord. At this point I decided to pay to have tests done on the cord and the placenta to make sure they were healthy and – guess what – they were fine.

I felt confident that my baby girl was just small and petite and everything was fine. However, the doctors needed to work to their hospital policies, which would mean inducing early for fear of the placenta not working. I would never have put my life or my baby's life in danger but I knew deep in my soul that my baby was well and I wanted and deserved to have the birth I'd dreamed of. Going into hospital would have been over-managed and would probably have ended up with intervention and drugs, which I didn't want for my precious baby just because she was small.

I later found out that the growth charts used by the hospital were based on European women and babies. However, if my husband had been the European and I had been Indian, my baby would have been classed as large.

After much thought we decided to go down the route of hiring an independent midwife. She came out to the house and spent many hours with us. She said she was happy to go ahead with our planned home birth and agreed that the baby was long and petite. At 37 weeks and 5 days, everything was set. For the next couple of weeks I had peace of mind.

When I awoke one Monday morning with period-like pains I wondered if this could be it. I had already lost part of my plug a few days earlier. By 9.30pm my contractions were stronger and closer together so my husband rang Sophie, our doula, to tell her and she said she was on her way.

When Sophie arrived I was in the lounge, leaning over a chair and breathing through each wave. The pressure was building and I knew my baby was going to arrive soon. After a short time my husband came up and said the pool was ready so I went downstairs to the room that I had set up; it felt so calm and peaceful. I moved slowly into the pool and the feeling and the warmth of the water really helped with each wave. I used only the warm water and breathing as pain relief and they both worked amazingly.

I spent the next hour just riding the waves of contractions with Sophie by my side talking me through each one. My husband was busy keeping the pool at the correct temperature and phoning the midwife. Helen the midwife arrived at 11.30pm and by this point I was into my stride, breathing through each wave. She checked the baby's heartbeat and monitored how dilated I was from the line on my lower back. I had asked for no internals unless it was necessary as I wanted to stay in the zone and keep the oxytocin flowing.

I had a very quick second stage of labour as I had breathed my baby all the way down using hypnobirthing breathing and meditation. Everyone was very surprised when she popped out into the water bright and alert after being in second stage for only 18 minutes. I scooped her up into my arms and couldn't believe my eyes when I realised I had a perfect little girl.

My little girl was small at 5 lb 11 oz but was strong, alert and perfect; my husband did skin to skin while I got out of the pool and delivered the placenta, as we knew we needed to keep her warm. We spent the next couple of hours upstairs in the lounge feeding her before we all snuggled up in bed together as a family. What an amazing day it had been. I'd had the most perfect birth and loved every minute.

My husband and I really did have an amazing birth. Having a doula and using hypnobirthing allowed me to have a wonderful, drug-free, enjoyable labour and birth.

LIVVI'S BIRTH

Livvi's mum used hypnobirthing techniques to overcome her fear of birth and have the home birth she wanted.

By Thursday 7 May I was nearly a week overdue and was starting to panic about not being able to have the home birth I desperately wanted. Thoughts of induction and hospital had started to enter my head. I felt really upset that I had done everything right – keeping active, walking with the dog every day – and still nothing was happening.

My partner Mike was supposed to have been going on a stag weekend on the Friday morning (planned before I was pregnant). We decided that we would see how I was on Friday afternoon and then think about him going just for a night. If labour did start he could be back within a few hours, and I would probably be in labour for a couple of days with my first baby.

I woke at 7.30am on Friday with regular but not painful contractions and knew that something was starting. I told Mike about the contractions but said I wasn't sure if it was just another false alarm. The problem was everyone had always told me you will feel it in your back and I didn't; my contractions were all at the front in my pelvis. We took the dog for a long walk and then at 10am Mike went to the pub to meet the lads before they left for the stag party. He would then make a decision late afternoon as to whether to join them or not.

By the time Mike left I knew this was it but thought I had a long way to go, and that I would probably have my baby by Sunday. So I set about some tasks, cleaning the house from top to bottom, taking the Tesco delivery and stocking the cupboards, having a bath and the most ridiculous task – doing my hair and putting on make-up! All the time the contractions were getting stronger and I was having to stop what I was doing and focus to get through them.

By 1pm I had to stop all tasks and focus on the contractions, which seemed so close together that there was no break between them. Mike was back and working on his laptop downstairs. I kept saying I needed him to finish, but by 1.30pm when he still wasn't done I went downstairs and virtually screamed at him that I needed him to stop and help me. I think that was probably the first time Mike thought it was really happening because until then I had been so focused and my usual self.

This phase was the only part of labour when I lost some of my control. The contractions were so intense and I allowed some doubt to enter my head as to whether I could do this. I think this was worsened by the fact that I always thought I would be able to find a comfy position to labour in and stick with it, but nothing was comfortable because my pain was so focused on my front. I had to be upright all the time and ended up moving around loads trying different positions, which I feel affected my ability to concentrate and focus.

Mike took control and put some chill-out music on. He helped me to visualise the Ibiza sunset I had used on the course to calm me through each contraction. He then called the hospital. The midwife and her trainee arrived at home just before 3pm. I had always said throughout my pregnancy that I didn't want to be examined in labour but I asked the midwife to examine me as I needed to know where I was.

The midwife told me I was over 5 cm dilated. That was the turning point for me. I had feared that I might not even be 1 cm, despite the intensity of the contractions, and was unsure I could cope with getting control back over my labour. Now I thought, 'I can bloody do this then!' It was like a whole wave of determination came over me. I got in the bath, which eased things for me. The midwives called for the gas and air, which in the end arrived too late to be of use. The hour or so in the bath seemed to pass so quickly but I was in control all of the time. It must have been funny to look at though because I was sitting bolt upright like on a high-backed chair, even though there was nothing behind me, because it was so uncomfortable to lie backwards.

When I said that I wanted to push at about 5.30pm the midwife was uncertain and wanted to check but then confirmed that I was ready. I was pushing by the time they called for a second midwife needed to deliver the baby. I remember thinking of the course at that moment and being told to trust your body. I had dilated 5 cm in just over two hours, which the textbook says couldn't happen!

I always thought that I would want to push by being upright kneeling forward but that just didn't work for me. I kept asking the midwives what to do and for advice but all the time felt totally in control like I was in charge and not them. My second midwife suggested I tried to push on the toilet, which helped just because I felt how to push and let myself do it properly, realising that I wasn't going to poo!

I wasn't comfortable on the toilet though, so after a couple of pushes I tried lying down and pulling my own knees which worked for me. Once I started pushing I felt so in control because I could feel what was happening with every contraction. I was really determined that I wasn't going to waste effort or a contraction. I found the physical feeling of having something to push against much easier than just sitting through a contraction. Again the whole thing went so quickly and in no time they said they could see her head. I was always really scared of this point, given what I had read about this being the most painful bit, but it wasn't.

I focused on what the midwives were telling me, giving small pushes and taking breaths as they were telling me so as not to tear. When her head came out they told me to rest but I said, 'No, I need to keep pushing,' and ended up pushing her out in one contraction. My beautiful baby girl was placed on my stomach at 6.38pm on Friday 8 May. I was just in total awe of her and speechless. I always thought I would be in floods of tears and had cried at every birth I had seen but I just lay looking at her while she grasped my hand.

Mike said later that he thought I had rejected her because I was so unemotional but I think I was just so focused on controlling the situation that it took me a while to come around. In my head it wasn't over until the midwives had gone and we were alone with our baby. It must have looked so odd but I sent Mike to call people and give the dog a quick walk while the midwife gave me a couple of stitches. By the time he returned I was tucked up in bed breastfeeding and they were getting ready to leave. By 8pm we were alone at home in our own bed just staring at our beautiful baby girl and that's when the emotion came for me. I didn't have to be in control any more; it was all done. The birth had been even better than I had imagined and we had made the most beautiful baby in the world.

Having the birth I wanted is the thing I am most proud of in my life. Thinking about it now makes me feel stronger and more confident as a person. I wish I could bottle the feeling! I know that I wouldn't have been able to do it without what I had learned. The hypnobirthing course enabled me to release the huge fear I had of childbirth and take control of my own birth experience, knowing that I had the inner strength to do it and the confidence to trust in my own body.

Some weeks later I played the CD again and remembered so much more about the birth. I hadn't consciously remembered the song Livvi was born to but as soon as it came on I burst into tears. Four months after she was born we took Livvi to see her very first Ibiza sunset for herself, and I hope that one day it will become her special place too.

GLOSSARY

Some of the terms mentioned in the book are listed below. There are also some others as it can be useful to have a quick reference for common terms that might crop up during your pregnancy and birth.

Beta-endorphins: The body's own natural painkillers, triggered by the increasing levels of oxytocin during labour. Their effects of pain relief and wellbeing resemble those of opiates such as pethidine, diamorphine and Meptid.

BMI: Your body mass index, a measure of body fat based on height and weight. If your BMI is over 30 you will be offered further tests for gestational diabetes and will be considered higher risk. However, just because you have a BMI of over 30, it doesn't mean that you will have a complicated pregnancy or birth. I have known women with a BMI of around 30 to have home births. The majority of pregnant women who have been categorised as obese due to their BMI go on to have perfectly normal births. Make sure that the person weighing you is accurate and that your individual circumstances are recognised.

Braxton Hicks: Contractions that are like warm-ups, getting you ready for labour. These can be quite regular sometimes, and can last a while. You may just notice your abdomen going hard or you may have to breathe through them. Not all women have them.

Cannula: A narrow tube used to administer a drip, antibiotics or fluids.

Cervix: The neck of your womb, and the gateway between your vagina and your womb. Did you know that birth is not the first time your cervix has dilated? Every time you have a period it dilates and your womb contracts. If you want to understand this more have a look at www.mybeautiful cervix.com. Women are undereducated about their bodies and this website is a great visual. You can also see how soft and expansive the tissues in that area of your body are. Someone once described the vagina as an accordion to me, and you can see how the soft ridging inside the vagina can help it expand and reduce in size.

Cord clamping: When the umbilical cord is clamped prior to cutting. You can have the cord clamped straight away or after two minutes. Alternatively, you can wait until it has stopped pulsating completely (delayed cord pulsation), which can take 10 minutes or longer. If the cord has stopped pulsating it does not need to be clamped as blood flow has ceased. In hospitals, staff may cut the cord quite early, though this is changing with strong evidence to show the overwhelming health benefits to baby of avoiding immediate cord clamping. Research has shown the benefits of delayed clamping with premature babies and even at Caesarean births.

CTG: A machine that continuously monitors your baby's heartbeat. This is routinely used if you are put on an oxytocin drip, or if you have an epidural, but also if your baby is considered to be compromised. If all is well, you can ask to be taken off it. You can also request long leads, which enable you to move about. Just because you are on a monitor does not mean that you have to stay on the bed. A patient midwife will help you move about. It is helpful to turn the sound off or down if it is a distraction. Research shows that continuous foetal monitoring does not always improve outcomes and can actually increase the risk of intervention.

Delayed cord pulsation: See 'cord clamping'.

Dilation: How your cervix softens and expands during labour. When it is 4–5 cm dilated you are considered to be in established labour. Dilation is sometimes expected to follow a curve, but remember that all women dilate in a different way. We dilate exponentially, which means the more we dilate the quicker it gets. You may get the urge to push at any time, maybe even a while after you are 10 cm dilated.

Doppler: A small electronic device that allows the midwife to listen to your baby's heartbeat. You will be familiar with them from your antenatal visits.

Doula: An additional birth partner hired by a couple to help support them emotionally and steer a course through labour that keeps to their birth preferences. Evidence shows that the presence of a doula can reduce the risk of a Caesarean birth by 50 per cent. Contact Doula UK to find out more (see Resources).

Established labour: In an actively managed model, established labour is considered to occur when the cervix is 4–5 cm dilated. There is much contention about this, though, as cervical dilation on its own is not an accurate predictor of when a baby will be born.

Ferguson reflex: The reflex that tells the body that baby is ready to be born. A mum often gets a strong urge to push at this point. I've heard mums say in retrospect that at this point their body just took over and all they had to do was let go.

First stage: The part of labour when your cervix is softening and dilating.

Induction: When labour is started artificially for one of many possible reasons. An induction can take the form of a drip or a pessary (see below). Avoid being scared into making a decision about induction. The hypnobirthing philosophy is to wait if all is well.

Limbic imprinting: How we make sense of the world around us so we can respond automatically. Many of our automatic responses are often laid down in our brain before we begin to talk. They continue to be laid down as we go through life, though on a slightly slower scale than through our formative years. Brain plasticity – the ability to alter patterns in the limbic system – has been shown to still be present in people in their 90s.

Membrane sweep: Often the first intervention in trying to get labour started. During a membrane sweep, your midwife will insert a finger into your vagina and feel for your cervix. She'll then sweep the cervix to separate the membranes from your cervix. A membrane sweep may be better closer to 42 weeks than 41 – most women are nearing labour at this point and it is more likely to be effective.

Neo-cortex: The part of your brain that thinks and is alert to logic, reason, time passing and self-awareness.

Oxytocin: Sometimes known as the love hormone, it is responsible for reproduction, birth and bonding. Oxytocin helps us birth by triggering the release of endorphins, and helps with the let-down reflex when breastfeeding.

Partogram: A record of the progress of labour, charting foetal heart rate, cervical dilation, blood pressure, pulse rate and so on.

Pessary: A tablet placed at the neck of the cervix which releases prostaglandins and can trigger labour. This is often the first step in an induction.

Physiological third stage: When the third stage of labour, after baby has been born, is left to run its course naturally. The body releases the placenta without any pharmacological help, responding to your own hormones. This usually takes under an hour but can sometimes be longer.

Second stage: The part of labour when your cervix is fully dilated and your baby begins to move down.

Syntocinon: The name for artificial oxytocin. It is usually given for an induction or to speed things up when contractions have slowed down or weakened. It may be given to help with the third stage instead of syntometrine (see below). Syntocinon does not cross the blood–brain barrier, and doesn't have the same effect as your own natural oxytocin in releasing endorphins. Sometimes you can go into labour naturally during an artificial induction. If you sense that this has happened, you can always ask for the drip to be turned down and then off. Some midwives will do this.

Syntometrine: Sometimes given to help the placenta release in the third stage after baby has been born. There is some evidence to suggest that it can negatively affect breastfeeding.

Transition: The moment when your body moves from first stage to second stage. Usually your cervix will be around 7–10 cm dilated. There is a shift in hormones from oxytocin to higher levels of adrenaline, and your contractions may come in waves. Sometimes, just before transition, there is a resting stage, or the 'rest and be thankful' stage. This can last for anything up to 30 minutes and can be a time when your body rests, contraction free, before your baby is born.

RESOURCES

BOOKS

Beaumont, Dean, *The Expectant Dad's Handbook* (Vermilion, 2013) – a very practical guide to birth for men

Buckley, Sarah, *Gentle Birth, Gentle Mothering* (Celestial Arts, 2009) – evidence-based work that can support your birth preferences, or encourage you to think about other things you may wish to include

Gaskin, Ina May, *Ina May's Guide to Childbirth* (Vermilion, 2008) – the book that most mums say changed their view of birth

Lokugamage, Amali, *The Heart is in the Womb* (Docamali, 2011) – written by a consultant obstetrician at a London hospital, this fantastic book explores what risk and decision making really mean. She herself was considered high risk because of her age and gestational diabetes

Ockwell-Smith, Sarah, *BabyCalm* (Piatkus, 2012) – will help you learn about your baby in those early days

Odent, Michel, *The Caesarean* (Free Association Books, 2004) – explores the rise of Caesarean birth, when it's necessary but also the potential overuse of it

Rapley, Gill and Murkett, Tracey, *Baby-led Breastfeeding* (Vermilion, 2012)

Simkin, Penny, *The Birth Partner* (Harvard Common Press, 2008) – this great little book explores possible emotional challenges that may come up during birth and explains what the mother is experiencing

Simkin, Penny, *Pregnancy, Childbirth and the Newborn* (Meadowbrook Press, 2010) – a comprehensive unbiased view of birth

INTERNET RESOURCES

doula.org.uk – for more information on doulas.

The Mindful Mamma blog (www.mindfulmamma.co.uk/blog) is always posting positive birth stories and evidence-based articles.

One World Birth (www.oneworldbirth.net) – a huge selection of short videos of midwives, doctors, doulas and mums talking about birth in a positive way. This is a great way of learning how your birth can be a positive experience.

'Tell me a Good Birth Story' (www.tellmeagoodbirthstory.com) is a wonderful project set up to encourage women to share positive birth stories. When you know other women have done it, you know you can do it too. Towards the end of your pregnancy, take time to read some of these stories.

ORGANISATIONS

AIMS (Association for Improvements in Maternity Services) – can provide information if you are concerned or made to feel frightened about your birth choices (www.aims.org.uk)

Association for Improvements in Maternity Care (AIMS) – publishes a set of leaflets on common questions that can arise. Good at supporting women to navigate their choices if they need help before the birth and are finding it difficult to get impartial advice (www.aims.org.uk)

Babycalm classes – parenting classes during pregnancy to prepare for those very early days of parenthood (www.babycalming.com)

Bliss – support for families of premature babies (www.bliss.org.uk)

La Leche League – breastfeeding support (www.laleche.org.uk)

National Childbirth Trust – support in pregnancy, birth and early parenthood across the UK (www.nct.org.uk)

NICE (National Institute of Clinical Excellence) – has clinical guidelines for standardised best practice across the UK. There are NICE guidelines for nearly every intervention in pregnancy (www.nice.org.uk)

Positive Birth Movement – groups helping support women to have positive births all over the UK (www.positivebirth.org)

ACKNOWLEDGEMENTS

First of all, thank you to my husband, Gordon, for his support in helping me do what I love. To Mia Scotland, whose insight and experience helped me set up Mindful Mamma, and who has been a gentle and thoughtful guide while I have been writing this book. Thanks to my mother, Jenny, whose wisdom and knowledge of mindfulness helped me reflect often on the techniques.

A guilty thanks to my children, Fin and Rory, who were handsomely rewarded for their patience after their summer holiday was taken up with edits.

Thank you to Julia Kellaway, without whom this book would still be languishing in a file on my desktop, to Louise Francis the commissioning editor who said yes, and to Sam Jackson, who taught me the importance and skill of a great editor. Thanks also to Nikki Syvret, Maureen Raynor, Nicky Grace, Marjory Fletcher and Stuart Flockhart, for proofreading, advice and rescue missions.

This book would not have been written without the input of all my Mindful Mamma practitioners who have supported me and contributed ideas. Thank you, you wonderful women. And, of course, a final thank you to all the couples whose stories are woven through the book and who have taught me what I'm just passing on.

INDEX

cord clamping 193, 203–4, 228, 229
corpus luteum 142, 143
cortisol 146
CTG 228–9

dates, going over your 199–200
delayed cord pulsation 193, 228, 229
diabetes, gestational 62, 219, 232
diamorphine 184, 227
diarrhoea 146
diet 147, 210, 219
different path, when things take a 194–204
dilation, cervical 105, 178, 184, 229, 230
Doppler 103, 229
doula 127, 134, 146, 183, 188, 189, 200–1, 229, 233
  birth choices and 94, 96, 107, 108
  birth space and 116, 117
  birth stories and 213, 219, 221, 222
  doula-led classes 74
  induction and 173
  midwife and 18, 165
  what's a? 89–91
Doula UK 90, 229
drug-free birth 3, 215, 222
drugs 3, 24–5, 56, 58, 180–1, 184–5, 204, 215, 220 *see also under individual drug name*

Entonox 184
environment, birthing *see* space/ environment, birth

epidural 74, 121, 134, 139, 152, 174, 176, 179, 180, 181, 185, 187, 203, 228
episiotomy 121
Erikson, Milton 30
established labour 152, 168–9, 229
exercises 4, 12–13, 15, 30, 32–3, 34, 37, 40, 44–9, 66–8, 75, 80, 83–4, 133, 136–7, 155, 160–1, 162, 190, 199–200, 210, 211

Facebook 73, 191, 192
fear and anxiety, letting go of 50–68
  creating your blank birth canvas 63–5
  expectation, anxiety, fear and pain 58–62
  hormones and 52–6
  how fear can slow down birth 56–7
  letting go of your fears 65–8
  your body and 51
Ferguson reflex 229
first birth 1, 56, 152, 200–1
first stage of labour 176, 229, 231
forceps 74, 102, 152, 174, 176, 180, 185
fourth stage ('babymoon') 207–8, 209

gas and air 184, 188, 203, 224
Gaskin, Ina May 69, 80–1, 232
Group B Strep (GBS) 93

hCG 143, 144